48·00

OSCE in Orthopedics

OSCE in Orthopedics

A Collection of Orthopedic Cases

S Kumaravel

MS (Ortho) D (Ortho) DNB (Ortho) PhD (Biomed Instrument)

Professor
Department of Orthopedics
Thanjavur Medical College
Thanjavur, Tamil Nadu, India

The Health Sciences Publisher

New Delhi | London | Panama

Jaypee Brothers Medical Publishers (P) Ltd

Headquarters

Jaypee Brothers Medical Publishers (P) Ltd
4838/24, Ansari Road, Daryaganj
New Delhi 110 002, India
Phone: +91-11-43574357
Fax: +91-11-43574314
Email: jaypee@jaypeebrothers.com

Overseas Offices

J.P. Medical Ltd
83 Victoria Street, London
SW1H 0HW (UK)
Phone: +44 20 3170 8910
Fax: +44 (0)20 3008 6180
Email: info@jpmedpub.com

Jaypee-Highlights Medical Publishers Inc
City of Knowledge, Bld. 235, 2nd Floor, Clayton
Panama City, Panama
Phone: +1 507-301-0496
Fax: +1 507-301-0499
Email: cservice@jphmedical.com

Jaypee Brothers Medical Publishers (P) Ltd
17/1-B Babar Road, Block-B, Shaymali
Mohammadpur, Dhaka-1207
Bangladesh
Mobile: +08801912003485
Email: jaypeedhaka@gmail.com

Jaypee Brothers Medical Publishers (P) Ltd
Bhotahity, Kathmandu
Nepal
Phone: +977-9741283608
Email: kathmandu@jaypeebrothers.com

Website: www.jaypeebrothers.com
Website: www.jaypeedigital.com

Inquiries for bulk sales may be solicited at: jaypee@jaypeebrothers.com

OSCE in Orthopedics

First Edition: **2017**

ISBN: 978-93-86322-13-5

Printed at: Samrat Offset Pvt. Ltd.

PREFACE

The book in your hands can very well be taken as a simple workbook on OSCE pattern of examination in orthopedics. I have used certain figures from our previous book *Short Cases in Orthopedics* as they deserve to be reiterated in OSCE model also. In an OSCE station, you can be given a clinical history, clinical finding investigation result, operative photographs, acute trauma photographs which one cannot be questioned in a regular (postgraduate or undergraduate) examinations. This book will familiarize this particular method to its readers. Although there are a few books available in the Western literature, this is the first of its kind exclusively written in India.

For decades, we have the evaluation method with different types of examiners. When the result arrives, the candidate who passed does not comment. When the candidate who does not pass, says one of the following:

- He got a tough case
- He was questioned severely
- He was failed though he did well
- The examiner was biased.

To debate and discuss whether the traditional system is best or OSCE is better is not the aim of this book. Traditional evaluation methods of the past are time tested but lack objectivity. When an examination method removes bias, standardize the patient and the examiner, then it makes only the candidate as the variable to be assessed.

There are a few steps to know how an OSCE is evolved:

1. First a clinical problem is written which can assess a candidate.
2. A method called the Sampling grid is applied to the above problem, i.e. exactly what is assessed in a candidate in that step (station).
3. Clear instructions are written to the candidate.
4. Similar instructions are also written to the examiner, patient or simulated patient.
5. A global rating sheet is written for the above problem giving weightage appropriately.
6. A list of items to be used in the station is written.
7. The OSCE problem is enacted.
   A key to any station or condition is what is the region and what is the lesion.

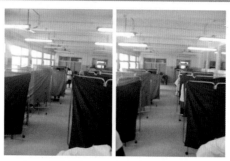

A serious OSCE examination is in progress

This book has more than 400 clinical cases with different types of questionnaires, and answers are given either as the written answer by the candidate or what is expected of him in such a situation. Both these are presented together. For the surprise factor which is normally seen in these types of examinations, I have mixed up the problems so that the mind of the student gets itself prepared. The onus in OSCE is on the examiners to set up an ideal OSCE with clean questioning. In that aspect, I really feel this book will be useful for them also.

This book can also be useful in such examinations like the PG-NEET, entrance examination of St. John's where OSCE like problem-oriented cases are discussed. This book will be effective **in regular theory examinations, especially writing a crisp short note,** both for undergraduates and postgraduates.

S Kumaravel

ACKNOWLEDGMENTS

The encouragement I received from my students for my first book *Short Cases in Orthopedics* published by M/s Jaypee Brothers Medical Publishers which was received with remarks *'Sir book semayya irrukku'* by my undergraduate and postgraduate students which means in colloquial Tamil 'Sir, the book is superb' urged me to work on to increase the number of illustrations in the present book. The clear difference between most of the books available in the market and this book in your hands is the sheer number of real patients shown in figures. I thank individual patients who were kind enough to co-operate. This collection of cases comes from 20 years of my personal work.

I thank my teachers Professor Mayil Vahanan Natarajan, Professor RH Govardhan, Professor CT Alagappan, Professor Nalli R Uvaraj, Professor R Selvaraj, Professor R Danapal, Professor K Chandran, and Professor M Sudheer, for all their interests in teaching me and making me what I am today.

I am very much indebted to Professor John Dent of Dundee, UK for having trained me in this aspect of medical education. I thank all my colleagues at Kilpauk Medical College, Thanjavur Medical College and Thiruvarur Medical College, DR Bharathy, Dr MS Manoharan, Dr V Jayapal, Dr P Venkatesan, Dr GA Rajmohan, Dr C Chinnadurai, Dr Thirumalaipandian, Dr Sivasenthil, and Dr Gopi. I thank my postgraduate students Dr Gobi Shankar Balaji, Dr N Karthikeyan, Dr M Manogaran, Dr Chandramohan, Dr C Karthikeyan, Dr T Angu, Dr Renjit John Mathew, Dr Mohamed Raheez, Dr Azath Faizer, Dr S Ashok, and Dr P Manigandan. I sincerely thank Prof Thiyaga Raja Sharma, for his advise and help in correcting the grammar of this book. I thank Miss N Bhuvaneswari of Bhuvana Infotech, Thanjavur for her help in bringing out corrections and placing the figures. I thank my physiotherapist Mr Muruganandam for all the help. I thank my parents Mr G Shanmugasundaram and Mrs Jayalaxmi Shanmugasundaram for the academic upbringing. I thank my better half, Dr Mangaleswari for all the help and my son Vishwa for all the encouragement.

I am also thankful to all the members in the production team of M/s Jaypee Brothers Medical Publishers (P) Ltd, New Delhi, India, for their constant support and cooperation in bringing out this book.

CONTENTS

Basics of OSCE

OSCE is objective structured clinical examination. The OSCE stations can be manned or unmanned. There can be real or simulated patients, i.e. volunteers, who can be used to tell symptoms like "I have knee pain for 10 months" etc

"The success of the result of the examination is in systematic method, concentrating on the process rather than the result."

In an ideal OSCE, the answer should be unambiguous and all students must see the same case. For critics of OSCE if one wants to differentiate an average student from a good performer, a specifically tough OSCE is the method. Lets us start with finding how an OSCE is formed with few examples. Rest of the book is a collection of OSCE based questions that can be from the cases seen in operation theaters, in ward rounds.

Instructions shall be given to the Candidate, Examiner and the Simulated patient
Example-1 -OSCE problem
35-year-old unconscious road accident victim brought to the casualty with his left lower limb splinted. What will a doctor receiving this patient do in the first 5 minutes?

Instructions shall be given to the Candidate

35-year-old unconscious road accident victim brought to the casualty. With his left lower limb splinted . You are the doctor receiving this patient what you will do in the first 5 minutes? What investigations you will order?

Instructions shall be given to the Simulated Patient

You are a 35-year-old unconscious road accident victim brought to the casualty with your left lower limb splinted. When the doctor examines and ask for anything don't respond by words or movement. You may be painted red with dye to simulate bleeding. Please cooperate.

Instructions shall be given to the Examiner

35-year-old unconscious road accident victim brought to the casualty. With his left lower limb splinted. The candidate is asked on receiving this patient, what will he do in the first 5 minutes? What investigations he will order?

Watch if the candidate looks for

1. Airway, breathing and circulation, cervical spine, pulses and BP.
2. Asks for suction airway oxygen IV fluids.
3. Assess Glasgow coma scale.
4. Looks for the limb injury.
5. Asks for whole body CT screening, X-rays of the leg and cervical spine lateral. blood grouping and electrolytes, sugar levels .

Example 2: Example of an OSCE

A hip problem patient can be given with malunited trochanteric fracture.

Instructions to the Candidate

This is a 45-year-old male presented after a fall and indigenous massage.
    Patient has a limp. He has pain in his left groin. Measure if he has a limb length discrepancy and in what segment?

Instructions shall be given to the Examiner

Please see if the candidate	Marks
1. Sees for the levels of anterior superior iliac spine	2
2. If left side is higher–squares the pelvis by carrying both the lower limbs together	2
3. Marks the bony landmarks of anterior superior iliac spine (ASIS), greater trochanter (GT), KJL, (knee joint line, medial malleolus (MM)	1
4. Measures from ASIS to KJL, KJL to MM	2
5. Draws Bryant's triangle	2
6. Measures the base of the Bryant's triangle	1

The same duration of **time** for all cases. There can be two stations based on the idea from **linked** and parallel stations. There need to be spare examiners and simulated patients. When one candidate is absent, in that slot the examiner fills that the candidate does not enter the **station**.

How will you measure the ability of a candidate? What is sampling grid?

A sampling grid is a measure of ability of a candidate. It is about what part of the candidate's ability is being examined. Sometimes, there can be an overlap of two ability in one test or station.
Marks weighting is done by competency for example

0=not demonstrated, ½= poorly demonstrated, 1= well demonstrated

		Expected outcome from candidate
Clinical skills	Demonstrating a clinical sign	Greets the patient Explains the test and gets permission
Practical procedures	Operations, Plaster applications Pin tractions	Lists 1. The indications 2. Requirements to perform the procedure 3. Tells what are the important precautions or structures to avoid
Investigations	Reading clinical report and X-ray	Tells the inference normal or wants further investigation
Patient management	Treatment	Tells the prognosis/says non-controversial answers.
Health promotion	Analyses the cause of the diseases and advises accordingly	In a case of genu valgum—rickets—the need for increased vitamin intake in siblings, to look for predisposing obstructive conditions. In a gastric carcinoma with bone secondaries advises siblings to undergo endoscopy
Communication	Delivering news of cancer, AIDS or death of a relative to the attenders	Make them sit Uses plain language, reinforces information Asks patient's concern ? Explain regarding nature of the disease The need to be positive in 1 and 2 And the tells about the amount of care given to the patient and in spite of all these the patient expired
Information handling	Data from a previous case record?	lists out the vital events of previous admission or out-patient treatment List outs the investigations that need to be repeated or not, etc
Basic clinical and social science	Analyses the strata of society that the patient comes from. The daily demand on his body especially joints	For a laborer he needs a stable hip. For a sedentary worker aggressive surgeries on the lateral ligament of ankle is not needed
Attitude and ethics	In case of a stage when the patient be preferably left alone uninvaded—it is better to leave him alone	Already established gastric carcinoma from gastric biopsy. If there is a bone secondaries, then no bone biopsy, is needed
Clinical judgment	On 4th day of an antibiotic, no response in infection. Wound has a greenish yellow discharge	You have to know it is due to *Pseudomonas* and start gram-negative bacteria specific antibiotics

Thus clinical skills, practical procedures, investigations, patient management, health promotion, communication, information handling, basic clinical and social skills, attitude and ethics, clinical judgment can be evaluated for any specific case.

The requirements of a particular station needs to be asked.

Venue	Osce 2013	Date				
Station	Description	Manned/ Unmanned	Examiner	Patient/ Simulated patient	Equipment needed	Marking sheet
1	Examination of an unconscious patient In first five minutes	Manned	Needed	Simulated patient	Personnel hall supervisor Nurse Timekeeper Answer sheets Cot, Two chairs Thomas splint Torch light BP apparatus Stethoscope Pulse-oximeter ECG monitor	

Itemized checklist.

Instructions to examiners

To observe how the candidate is going about to evaluate an unconscious patient:

No need to greet

1. Candidate must be able to assess GCS
   The following must be evaluated:
   Able to tell EMV—Able to explain sub classification of EMV
2. Assessment of the ABCC
3. Looks for chest and abdominal injuries
4. Looks for the limb injury
   ◊ Investigation, he needs to order
   ◊ Trauma series X-rays -Skull, cervical spine, chest and pelvis
   ◊ Whole body CT scan
   ◊ Steps in management
   ◊ Management of head injury,
   ◊ Management of intra-abdominal or thoracic injury
   ◊ Management of limb injury
   ◊ Inform immediate supervisor or consultant.

Instructions to the simulated patient

You are Mr. X; you are supposed to be an RTA victim who is unconscious with a fracture in your right leg. Do not respond to any verbal commands and any painful stimuli just sleep. Your right leg will be splinted.

Instructions to the candidate

At this station you will be asked to answer the following question

- You are a resident on call
- You get a 30-year-old unconscious patient with a closed tibial fracture on a splint

Sampling Grid

Out Come	Clinical skills	Practical proce-dures	Investig ations	Patient man-agement	Health promotion	Commu-nication	Inform ation handling	Basic clinical and social science	Attitude and ethics	Clinical judgement
Manned	+	+	+	+		+				+
Un manned										

- You are required to explain what you are doing as you do
- Assess his unconsciousness?
- What will you assess next?
- What are the imaging you will perform?
- What is the sequential step of management?
- After evaluation and resuscitating what will be your next step.

Examiners checklist

You are about to discharge a patient who had a hemiarthroplasty for a fractured neck of femur. Patient with a dressing is done in the hip region.

What are the points you will tell the patient?.   Marks

1. Greeting the patient.   1
2. Tells about the type of the hip cemented or uncemented.   1
3. Advises to keep the leg abducted with a knee brace.   1
4. Advises walking with a walker.   1
5. Advises not to take bath and keep the dressing dry till
   next visit.   1
6. Not to keep the legs cross.   1
7. Advises to move the ankle and do static quadriceps
   setting exercises.   1
8. Report any ooze and bleeding from the dressing.   1
9. Report any swelling of the calf.   1
10. Continue anti-clotting medication and pain relief
    medications as advised.   1

We shall see a few other examples.

Problem 1. Instruction to the Candidate

- Identify the lesion—a picture of wrist drop is displayed
- Write the structures involved in the pathogenesis of this condition?
- Write the commonest site of lesion.
- Write all the branches of the structure at that level.

Instruction to the Examiner	**Marks**
If candidate tells	
Wrist drop	1
Radial nerve	1
Spiral groove	1
• 2 muscular branches–N to medial head of triceps, N to lateral head of triceps	½ + ½
• 2 cutaneous branches- posterior cutaneous nerve of forearm and lower lateral cutaneous nerve of arm	½ + ½

Problem 2. Intramedullary reamer for ILN:

- Identify the instrument
- What are the indications and contraindications?

Problem 3. A histopathology slide is given ?

Pain over the sternum.

- What is the diagnosis? Further investigations. What is the drug of choice? What other organ it affects?
- Slide of plasma cell tumor.
- Whole body Tc 99 scan
- Melphalan.
- Kidneys.

Problem 4. An X-ray of heel.

Pain over the heel. More in the morning and reduced. What is the diagnosis? Further investigations.
- Plantar fasciitis
- X-ray of both heels lateral view
- Uric acid
- Blood sugar.

Problem 5. A 12 year old boy had a fracture elbow with severe swelling of forearm. Finger movements are reduced and painful. What is the diagnosis?

- Compartment-syndrome.
- How will you objectively assess this condition?
- By measuring compartment pressure.

Problem 6. Bone cement.

- What is this ampoule and sachet?
- Bone cement.   1
- What are its components? Polymer and monomer   1
- Indications of its use.
- Fixing an implant, augmenting a fixation and filling a cavity after curettage of benign bone lesion, Vertebra plasty.   ½ each.
- Side effects of this?
- Spillage into surroundings   ½ each.
- Hypotension.

Problem 7.

- Hypocalcemic tetany
- 30-year-lady underwent neck surgery has developed the following features the next day of surgery.

Instruction to Candidate
- What is the diagnosis? What is the etiology?

Instruction to Examiner
- Look if the candidate examines the limbs
- Whether gives the answer as hypocalcemia
- Hysterical respiratory acidosis.

Instruction to Simulated Patient
- To keep the limb in a position of carpopedal spasm.   Marks
- If the candidate tells Acouchier's hand.
- Carpopedal spasm   3
- Two causes
- Hypocalcemia   1
- Hysterical respiratory acidosis   1

Problem 8

1.5-year-old male child brought to the casualty with not using his left upper limb since afternoon.
- There is no gross swelling of the arm elbow or forearm. X-rays are normal.
- Management of the case.
- Investigations required for the patients.
- What are the questions you will ask? The candidate ask for who looks after the child?
- What violence will you ask? Pulling by an older child or house maid.

Problem 9

35-year-old female patient with multinodular goiter with toxic features fell and had a tibial fracture.
Instructions to Candidate.
- Name three important peroperative advice/instructions to the patient/history you will ask?
Instructions to Examiner
- Ask if candidate asks.
1. Antithyroid drugs,
2. Post operative voice change,
3. Symptoms of hypocalcaemia.
- Name one examination which will mark the control of the disease?
- Sleeping pulse rate.
- What is the problem in operating on this lady?
- The operation may get delayed for control of the toxicity.

Problem 10

55-year-gentleman has LBA with dysuria.
- What are the questions you will ask?
- Asks duration of symptoms and gives probable system diagnosis.
- What are the investigations you will order?
- Basic investigations what to look for.
- Special investigations based on basic investigation and clinical conclusions.

Instructions to Simulated Patient
- You are Mr. X with LBA for 4 months and difficult in micturition for 1 year. You have weakness of both lower limbs for 1 month. Thanks for your cooperation.

Instructions to Candidate
- Ask about the symptoms.
- Ask about the patient regarding relevant additional questions.
- Prostrate swelling- any irritation during voiding, any incomplete emptying.
- Weaknessà find it difficult to walk without support.
- Secondaries—diffuse pain in the back.

Problem 11

60-year-old lady who fell down and had a fracture of upper humerus. She had a small contusion over the left temporal region. Her CT scan of brain is given. (Showed multiple altered intensities in the occipital lobes and on right lung field adjacent to her right shoulder). She was operated for cancer right breast 11 months back.
- Identification of abnormal lesions 2 ½
- What is the possible diagnosis?
- Secondaries in lungs and brain
- Differential diagnosis. 2 ½

Problem 12

Unmanned Station

26-year-old Mr. K presented to the hospital with diffuse crush injury to his right leg. One week before he had fever and vomiting for 3 days.
- O/E Febrile, vitals stable, r/e crepitations right leg region, X-rays are displayed.

Instructions to Candidate
- What is the clinical diagnosis?
- Gas gangrene.
- Differential diagnosis.
- Cellulitis.
- X - ray findings.
- Gas in the soft tissue.
- Differential diagnosis.
- Final diagnosis.
- How will you manage?
- Debridement, Amputation.
- Anti gas gangrene serum.

Problem 13

Rickets

Instructions to Candidate
- What is this disease?
- Is it prevalent in India?
- How does it happen?
- How can this disease be prevented?

Problem 14

Unmanned Station

A 45-year man came with a swelling and pain over the right greattoe.

- There is no other site of pain.
- What is the possible diagnosis?
- What history of diet will you like to ask?
- What are the foodstuffs you need to avoid?
- What is the biochemical investigation you will order?

Problem 15

A 39-year-old male presented with stiff back with severe stiffness in the morning. Had redness of the eye and photo phobia.

- What is the possible diagnosis?
- Ankylosing spondylitis.
- What blood investigations apart from ESR are useful in pinning the diagnosis?
- HLA-B27.
- Name one region you will order an X-ray for diagnosing the lesion. X-ray lumbosacrum.
- What possibly happened to his eyes?
- Iridocyclitis.

■ SUGGESTED READING

1. Collins JP, Harden RM AMEE Medical Education GN13, real patients, simulated patients and simulators in clinical examinations. Medical Teacher. 1998;20(6): 508-21
2. Harden RM, Stevenson M, Downie WW, Wilson GM. Assessment of clinical competence by objective structured examinations. BMJ. 1975;447-51
3. Instructional course lectures by Prof John Dent, In Dr MGR Medical University, Chennai on 3rd and 4th December 2010.
4. Objective clinical structured examination(OSCE) revisited. J Posgrad Med Education, Training and Research 6 2009;1-10
5. Selby C, Osman L, Davis M, Lee M. Setup and run an objective structured clinical exam, . BMJ. 1995;310:1187-90.

Model OSCE Problems Part 1

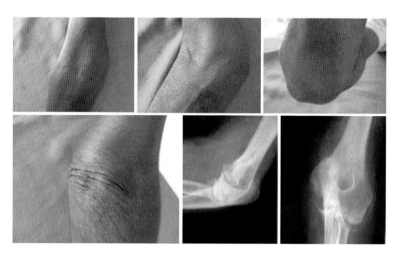

Instructions given to the Candidate.

This 30-year-old lady came with a swelling of right elbow without much pain.

What is the possible diagnosis?

Neuropathic joint.

What is the probable cause of this painless swelling?

What is the region of the possible primary lesion?

What is the lesion?

• Syringomyelia of the cervical spine.

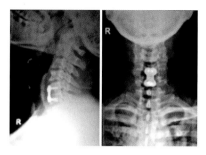

Instructions given to the Candidate

What are the precautions for applying the screws as to the direction of screws?

Screws are applied to avoid vertebral arteries in the medial superior direction.

What are the structures to be avoided?

- Avoid vertebral arteries.

These screws are uni-cortical only. Is it ok? How?

- Yes, they are locking screws.

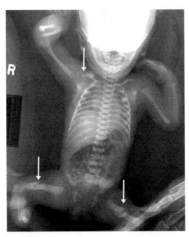

This 1 day old neonate was brought to you without any history of injury. What is your opinion of the pointed arrows?

When the event causing the lesion should have happened?

Right clavicle and left femur should be intrauterine.

Right femur fresh fracture.

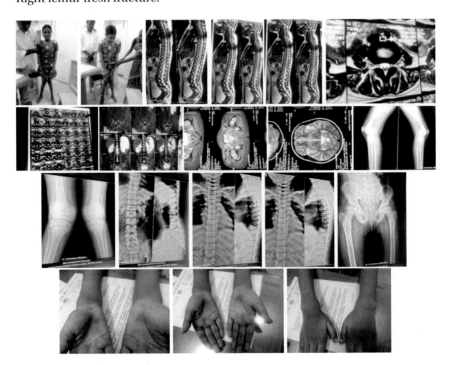

Instructions given to the Candidate

A 13-year-old girl found it difficult to get up and walk for past 6 months. These are her spine knee X-rays. Serum calcium, Phosphorus, Alkaline phosphatase and Parathyroid hormone were normal. Bilateral medical renal disease with grade 2 disease with corticomedullary thickness. lower limit normal. MRI is normal

What is the possible diagnosis?

Rickets

What is the posible cause?

Renal rickets

How will you treat her?

High dose vitamin D and calcium

Will you correct the deformity ? When?

When the patient is adequately treated with high dose vitamin D and calcium and healed well.

What is the possible differential diagnosis?

Proximal muscle weakness

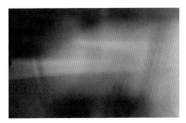 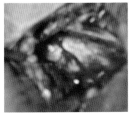

Distal proximal   Distal proximal

Instructions given to the Candidate

On your left, you have the X-ray of the shaft of femur
On the right, you see a plate being placed over the same fracture (on the table)

Which screw will you apply first and why?

Distal

The obliqueness will hold the proximal spike along with the plate.

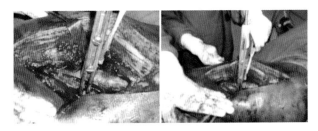

Instructions given to the Candidate

What is being done?

An oblique fracture being reduced.

What is this instrument?
Lowman's clamp.

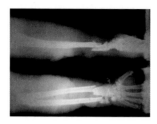

Instructions given to the Candidate

What injury do you see?
What is your opinion about the soft tissue component?
Fracture both bones of fracture with soft tissue injury.

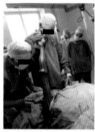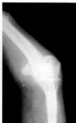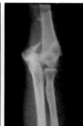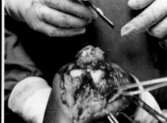

Instructions given to the Candidate

What is this fracture?
Supra condylar fracture with intercondylar extension

What is this approach seen in last figure is called?
Campbell's posterior approach

How will you fix this fracture?
By fixing the inter-condylar element first followed by re-constructing both the columns.

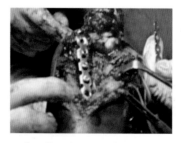

This is the same fracture after fixation.

What is the implant used?
Reconstruction plate.

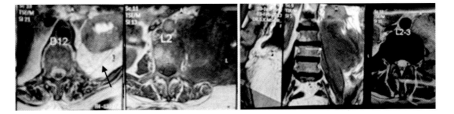

Instructions given to the Candidate

This 65-year-old lady presented with a draining sinus on the left loin. What do you look on the left side of vertebral bodies in these films (arrow-pointing to which lesion)?
Peri-nephric collection of fluid/pus.

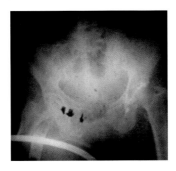

Instructions given to the Candidate

What is the orthopedic injury? Subtrochanteric fracture
Name the accepted classification of this fracture ?
Russel-Taylor-type A2 piriformis fossa intact and lesser trochanter fractured.

What is the AO classification of this fracture?
AO has not classified this fracture.

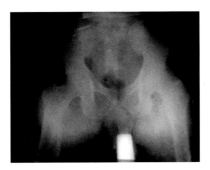

Instructions given to the Candidate

What is this fracture?
Sub-trochanteric fracture.

What is the implant of choice?
Reconstruction nail.

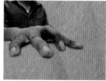 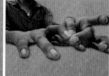 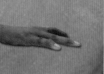 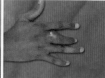

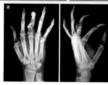

Instructions given to the Candidate

This 25-year-old had a fall of a sharp machinery part onto his right hand at his work place.

What has happened?

The patient's middle finger is stiff and deformed.

Fracture proximal phalanx with bone loss.

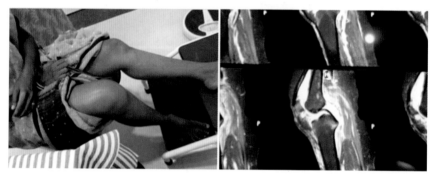

Instructions given to the Candidate

This 35-year-old lady came with gross pain and swelling of her right knee with this picture for 4 month duration. Her MRI is shown.

What do you see in her MRI?

Soft tissue swelling with synovial effusion.

What are the other serological tests you will order?

Tests for TB and Rheumatoid Arthritis, reactive arthritis must be done.

How will you treat the patient till results arrive?

The knee is immobilized.

Analgesics given according to her pain.

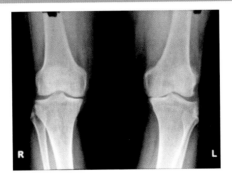

What is the view?
Standing Anteroposterior views.

What is your diagnosis?
Degeneration with varus deformity.

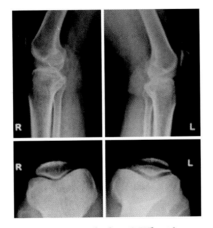

What is the name of the view seen below? What is seen in the lower view?
What is your diagnosis?
Skyline view.
Patellofemoral arthritis.

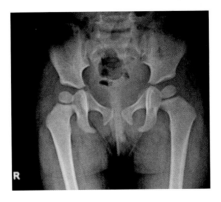

What is the age of this child?
Prepubertal.
Why?
Ilium is formed at 2nd month, ischium at 3rd month and pubis at 5th month of intrauterine life.
Head is formed – 6 months to 1 year extrauterine life
In the X-ray not formed are ischial tuberosity and symphysis pubis, iliac crest (Riser's sign) → hence child not reached puberty.

What are the orthopedic significance?
Child is skeletally immature- hence prone for progressive spinal deformity.

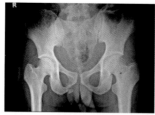 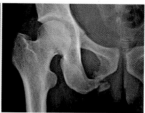

Instructions given to the Candidate

What are the orthopedic injuries in this pelvis?
Fracture of acetabular floor
Inferior pubic rami fracture.

What other investigations you will order to manage this condition?
CT scan of pelvis.

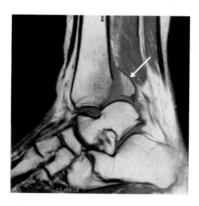

Instructions given to the Candidate

What is this injury?
Posterior malleolus fracture with a subluxed ankle.

How will you treat this condition?
Usually associated with medial and lateral malleoli fracture and they are first treated and the posterior malleolus is fixed (especially if more than 25% of the articular surface are involved).

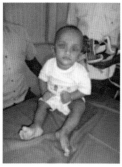 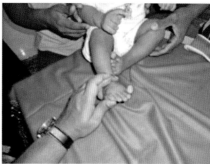

Instructions given to the Candidate

What is being attempted in the second picture?
Forefoot is pronated.
What is this condition?
Club foot (CTEV).

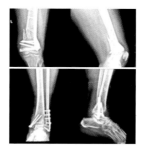

Instructions given to the Candidate

All these X-rays belong to one single patient.

What are the probable orthopedic injuries in knee and ankle?
Distal femoral fracture/bimalleolar fracture.

What are the implants used?
For distal femur fracture, condylar buttress plate; Plate and screws for fibula and cancellous screws for medial malleolus.

A 12-year-old boy presented with swelling and pain in the lower leg. Patient did not have any constitutional symptoms. (see figures below)

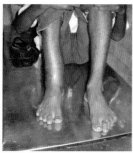 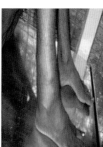 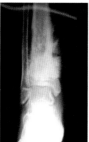 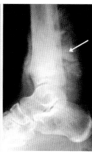

What is the possible diagnosis you can tell?

It is a malignant bone tumor most probably it may be Osteosarcoma.

How to suspect this tumor clinically?

Onset in 1st and 2nd decade; No joint involvement (may have extra-articular restriction); No constitutional symptoms.

What will you look for in the X-ray of the part?

- Periosteal elevation
- Bone destruction
- Cortical erosion
- Pathological fracture
- Soft tissue involvement in the form of calcifications.

How the pointed structures are formed?

They are the Sunray spicules. They are formed along the blood vessels of periosteum as it is elevated or hypothesized to be formed by the Sharpey's fibre of the periosteum

What is the next investigation for local staging in this condition?

MRI.

How is this condition staged for treatment?

Enneking stage — IA → Intracompartmental- low grade - plan Limb salvage

IB → Extracompartmental -low grade – Ablation

IIA → Intracompartmental -high grade - Limb salvage

IIB → Extracompartmental -high grade – Ablation

III → Metastasis- Palliative ablation/chemotherapy/ Radiotherapy.

How will you confirm the disease? What bearing the biopsy site have over treatment ?

Since OS patients should be approached positively, i.e with chemotherapy they live longer. We should not hamper that chance of limb salvage. Better a core needle biopsy where dissemination chance is less and if needle specimen is inadequate, open incisional biopsy is planned so that the scan with margin is removed in definitive surgery.

In the following case of a malignant tumor of the lower femur, where will you take the biopsy from?A, B or C?

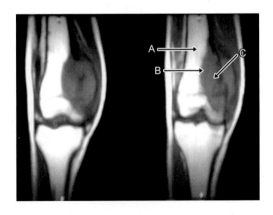

The junction of normal and tumor tissue.

Any other important factor other than stage and adequacy of resection ?

Yes. Tumor size. Smaller the tumor better is the prognosis.
The tumor's response to chemotherapy is also better.
Tumor necrosis after chemotherapy is the only significant variable

What is classical picture of this tumor ?

Metaphysis, Codman's triangle, Sunray spicules, no pathological fracture.

General Questions

What are the components of limb salvage?

Wide excision of the tumor followed by reconstruction.
In adults, knee joint fusion, endoprosthesis, allograft, ilizarov, rotation plasty.
In children expandable prosthesis

Name 5 advantages of Neo-adjuvant chemotherapy.

1. Controls micrometasis and metastasis during surgery.
2. Tumor regression.
3. Decrease vascularity.
4. Tumor becomes hard and easy to dissect.
5. It gives time to prepare custom prosthesis for the size of the patient's bone.
6. Chemotherapy given before surgery, the resected specimen can be sent for study of necrotic material and chemotherapeutic drugs can be changed if no necrosis.

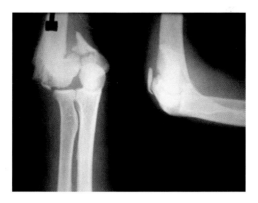

Instructions given to the Candidate

What is this injury? How will you treat this fracture?

Intercondylar fracture of humerus with supracondylar extension.
This should be operated by:
1. Fixing the intercondylar fracture parts into one fragment.
2. Fixing this composite fragment to the shaft by plates.

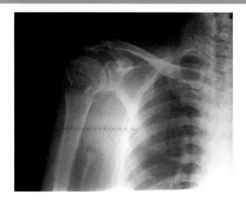

Instructions given to the Candidate

This is the X-ray of a 55-year-old diabetic male.

What are the orthopedic injuries?
Proximal humeral fracture.

How will you investigate this injury?
Reconstruction CT scan.

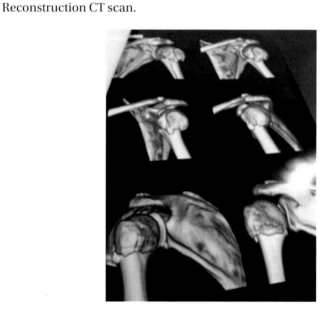

Instructions given to the Candidate

This is the reconstruction CT of the above patient.
What is the injury?
How will you proceed?
Displaced four part fracture.
Hemiarthroplasty.

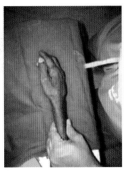 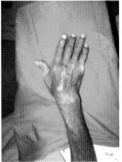

Instructions given to the Candidate

What is the orthopedic injury?

Carpometacarpal dislocation

How will you manage?

X-ray confirmation.

Closed or open reduction and K –wire fixation.

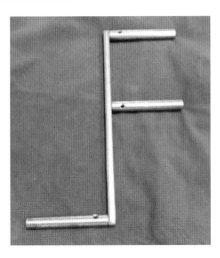

What is this instrument? How it is fitted? What are its uses?

There is a centre bar on either side of which there are threaded holes which allow fitting the threaded rods in position. Two threaded rods are placed on one side and one on the other side as seen in the above figure. The threaded rods reduce the fractures and also hold the reduction till the guide wire or the ender nail is introduced. After the surgery the parts can be disassembled and cleaned.

For which side this instrument is used right or left?

They can be used in both side limbs.

What is the metal it is made of? Is it radiolucent?

It is made of aluminium and is not radiolucent.

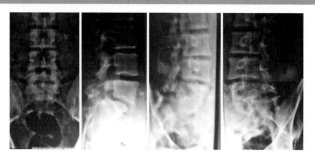

Instructions given to the Candidate

What do you see in first two figures?
Routine AP and lateral views of lumbosacral spine.

What are these views next two figures?
Right and left oblique views of lumbo sacral spine.

What is the need for these last two views ?
To find any pars interarticular defect.

What is the classical appearance of this problem seen in the above special views?
Beheaded Scottish Terrier appearance/Lysis is seen.

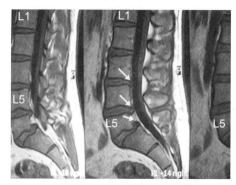

This is the MRI of a patient with leg pain on walking only
He does not have any neurologic deficit on clinical examination
What is your diagnosis?
Neurogenic claudication.

Why this lesion affects only lower lumbar and sacral roots?
Because lower intervertebral foramina are progressively smaller.

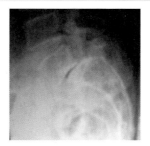

What is this condition?
Spondylolisthesis LS/S1

What is the grade?
Grade 2 listhesis

What is the treatment?
Pelvic -traction for 6 weeks.

When will you operate?
If pelvic traction did not relieve the pain.

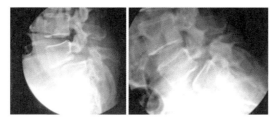

What are these two views?
Extension and Flexion views

What is the possible lesion?
Spondylolisthesis.

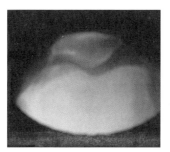

What is this X-ray?
Skyline view of the knee.

What is the finding in the X-ray?
Patella femoral arthritis.

What will be the two main activities that will become restricted by this condition?
Climbing stairs and squatting.

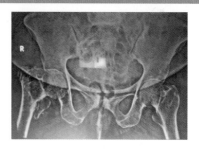

This an 80-year-old lady had a fall.

What is the lesion?
Inter-trochanteric fracture on the right side.

What is the type of the lesion?
Type 2 Boyd and Griffith.

What is the preferred treatment?
Cemented hemiarthroplasty.

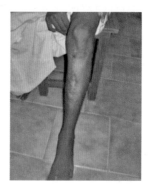

This 45-year-old man came with pain in a previously operated area (25 years back) over the left leg. He had mild elevation of his temperature and ESR.

What shall be your diagnosis?
Reactivation of old osteomyelitis

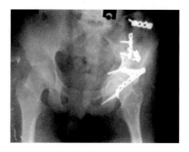

This 23-year-old came with this procedure done elsewhere.

What shall be the original fractures?
Acetabular fracture with 2 column involvement.

What are the implants used?
Reconstruction plate and cancellous screws.

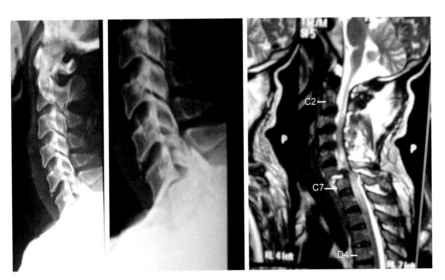

What is the level lesion?
C6/7.

What is the lesion?
C6/7 listhesis.

What is the possible outcome of such an injury?
Quadriparesis.

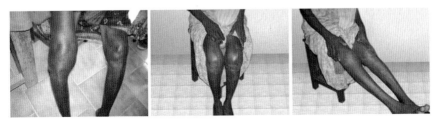

First is a preoperative status, second and third are postoperative status.
What is the diagnosis of this case?
Bilateral genu varum – Osteoathritis knee.

What is the possible surgery done?
Total knee arthroplasty.

What is the preoperative measurement to be done?
Inter condylar distance.

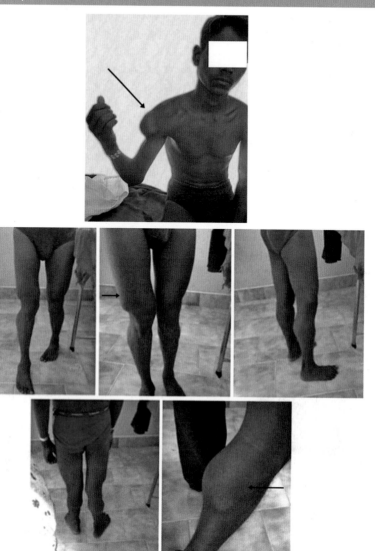

A young male came with multiple swellings of right upper arm, right femur right tibia.

What is the diagnosis?

A case of multiple exostosis of right upper arm, right femur and right tibia.

What are the lesions you will operate ?

The symptomatic exostosis will be removed.

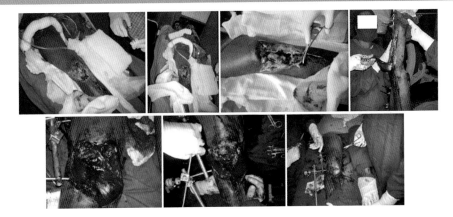

Instructions given to the Candidate

A 50-year-old male had upper tibial fracture. You are seeing preoperative and intra operative photographs.

What is the diagnosis from the snaps seen in 1st 3 photos?
Upper tibial fracture with soft tissue injury.

What are the procedures seen in next 3 photos?
External fixator application and muscle flap—medial gastrocnemius flap.

What is the procedure seen in last snap?
SSG over the above flap site.

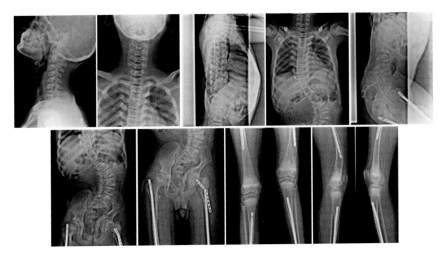

Instructions given to the Candidate

All these are X-rays of an 11-year-old, who has been operated for a condition.

What is the diagnosis?
Osteogenesis Imperfecta with Spinal deformities

What are the procedures done?
Prophylactic fixations with nails and plating.

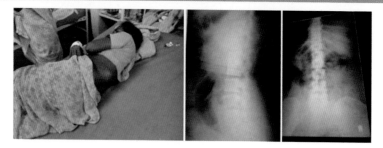

Instructions given to the Candidate

This is a 45-year-old lady with this finding. Other 2 figures are her X –rays.

What is the swelling ?

Cold abscess

What is the possible cause?

Cold abscess –tuberculous.

How this lesion tracks?

Cold abscess tracks along the intercostal and cutanoeous nerves.

What are the serological investigations you will order?

TB ELISA, TB-PCR.

What are the further imaging you will do?

MRI spine.

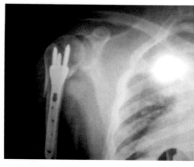
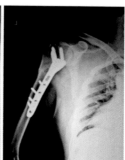

Instructions given to the Candidate

This is the X-ray of a 25-year-old gentleman who was operated for a fracture upper humerus?

What is the implant used?

Locking compression plate for proximal humerus.

What is the (prerequisite for) step necessary before applying this implant?

Reduction of the fracture

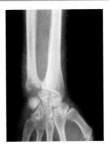

This is a 50-year-old gentle man who had pain wrist for past 3 years, with loss of appetite and weight. His X-ray showed this finding.

What are the differential diagnosis?

Lytic lesion of distal ulna.

Tuberculosis of the distal ulna.

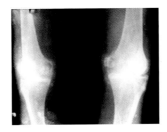

Instructions given to the candidate

This is a 50-year-old lady who had pain both knees for past 5 years . Her X-ray showed this finding.

What is the differential diagnosis?

Osteoarthrosis of the knee joints, pseudogout, and ochronosis

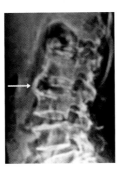

Instructions given to the Candidate

What is the pointed structure?

Syndesmophyte.

Name one condition which causes this?

• Ankylosing spondylitis.

What is the structure which forms this?

Annulus fibrosis.

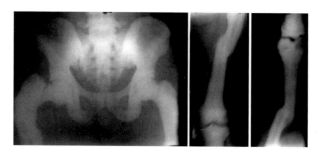

Instructions given to the Candidate

All these are X-rays of a 45-year-old,

What is the radiological finding of these bone in general apart from the fractures?

There is no cortical and medullary differentiaton.

What is the diagnosis?

Marble bone disease with neck of femur fracture and shaft of femur fracture.

What will be their calcium and alkaline phosphate levels?

Usually normal.

What are the problems?

Fixations with nailing and plating are difficult.

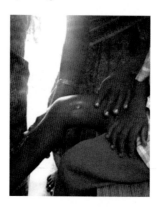

This 14-year old has pain over lower thigh and fever. What is the possible diagnosis?

Osteomyelitis of lower femur.

Preferable knowledge to have on the natural course of this condition.

Sinus with discharge-Growth disturbance – Pathological fracture deformity.

What are the 3 main palpatory examinations you will do and how will you do it?

Greet, Explain, get consent and undress patient.

{The candidate} He will feel

- Warmth in the region Normal side first –lesion side next and normal side again.
- Thickening of bone Normal side first –lesion side for comparison.
- Tenderness- is seen by pressing on the site of lesion and seeing observing the face of the child for any possible grimace or reaction.
- Shortening /lengthening is measured
- Lymphnoe palpation.

Definition this condition?

Osteomyelitis is inflammation of bone and marrow (usually blood borne).

Why in metaphysis?

1. Vascularity and hairpin loop of capillaries—causes slowing of blood.
2. Macrophage activity is less.

What are the stages of this disease?

Intramedullary abscess → Subperiosteal abscess → Stripping of the periosteum → Diaphyseal sequestrum → Periosteum forming new bone called involucrum.

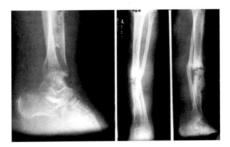

Instructions given to the Candidate

What has happened to the fibula?

It is angulated

Will this will affect the length of the bone?

Shortens the tibia.

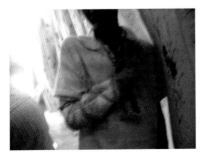

Instructions given to the Candidate

This boy was immobilized with a plaster.
What has happened to the plaster?
The boy has broken the plaster.

What is the possible diagnosis for which plaster is applied?
Contusion elbow
Operated and internally fixed case allowing movement.

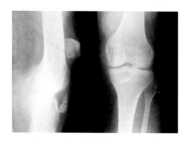

Instructions given to the Candidate

What is the diagnosis? Patella feacture-nonunion
What will be the clinical finding? Patient cannot do straight leg raising
How will you incise for the surgery?
Longitudinal midline incision.

What are the treatment options available?
Tension band wiring.

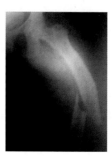

Instructions given to the Candidate

In this X-ray of femur what do you observe?
What is needed before concluding on management?
Excessive bowing with fracture of femur
X-ray of the knee and pelvis should be included to rule out other injuries.
X-ray of opposite side femur to rule out pathology.

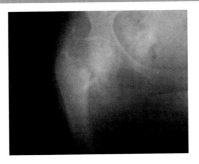

Instructions given to the Candidate

This is an X-ray of a 50-year-old female

What is this lesion?
Fracture neck of femur.

What other special X-ray view will you order and why?
Traction and internal rotation view to assess the availability of calcar.

What are the other imaging studies that will be useful?
MRI of pelvis.
Tc 99 scan of the pelvis.

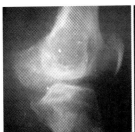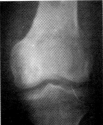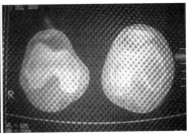

Instructions given to the candidate

30-year-old lady came with 6 month pain over left knee and inability to walk for past 1 month.

Diagnosis
GCT femoral condyle

What are the immediate local problems it can cause in this case?
Pathological fracture.

What is the type of the lesion and why?
Since there is no sclerosis around the lesion, it must be an aggressive lesion.

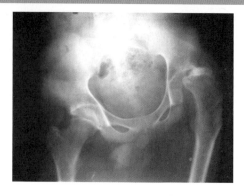

Instructions given to the Candidate

What is the lesion in the left hip? Perthes disease
Is there any risk sign?
Horizontal epiphysis.
Sclerosis of the head.
What are the treatment options available?
Varus derotation osteotomy.
Replacement at a later stage.

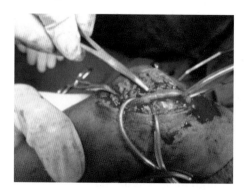

Instructions given to the Candidate

This is a surgery done in a child for her elbow injury.
What is the structure which is protected by the infant feeding tube?
Ulnar nerve

What test you will do to check post operatively regarding any iatrogenic injury?
Sensation over tip of the little finger and
Intrinsic muscle action.

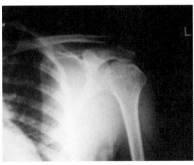 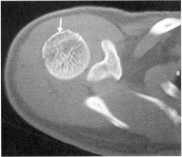

Instructions given to the Candidate

What is the diagnosis?

Greater tuberosity fracture with a large fragment of bone with minimal displacement.

A 2-part fracture.

What are the treatment options available?

Internal fixation with cancellous screws (or) conservation.

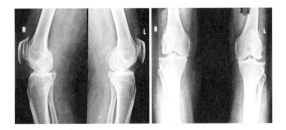

Instructions given to the Candidate

What are the joints involved?

Patello-femoral and medial compartment more involved.

Is there a chance for high tibial osteotomy?

No.

What are the options of treatment?

If conservation fails → Total knee arthroplasty.

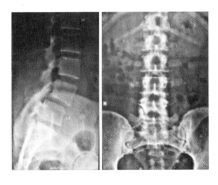

Instructions given to the Candidate

What is the diagnosis (from the above X-ray)?
L4/5 listhesis.

What will be the clinical finding?
Pain at concerned side lower limb and weakness of Extensor Hallucis Longus in the same side

What are the options available?
Traction and if no relief, discectomy and fusion.

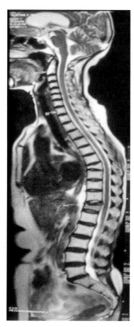

A 75 year old lady had spontaneous back pain with difficulty in even turning to sides. Her MRI is shown above. Locate the lesions?
D8 and D12

What type of lesion are these?
Anterior wedge compression fractures.

From the available picture can you tell which lesion happened first? Why?
D7 happened first and D12 recently-because of marrow edema in D12.

Which lesion is causing the pain now?
D12 fracture.

How will you treat this non-invasively?
Spinal braces, Calcitonin spray, Oral calcium, Rest

Is there any method of treating it invasively?
Vertebroplasty

Instructions given to the Candidate

What is the obvious lesion in spine?
Lysis of L5.

What will be the clinical finding?

Mechanical pain on stooping forward.

What are the initial treatment options available?

Pelvic traction and spinal extension exercises.

If pain persists after conservative treatment what will you do?

Fusion.

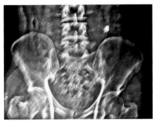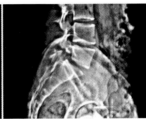

Instructions given to the Candidate

What is the diagnosis?

Lysis of L5.

What will be the clinical finding?

Mechanical pain on stooping forward.

What are the options available?

Pelvic traction and spinal extension exercises

If pain persists what will yo do?

Fusion.

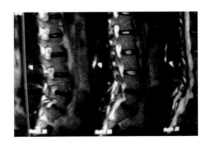

Instructions given to the Candidate

What is the diagnosis?

Intervertebral disc prolapse.

What will be the clinical finding?

Pain in the leg usually unilateral

What are the treatment options available?

Physiotherapy, NSAIDs, Pregabalin
Discectomy and Fusion.

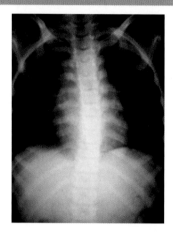

Instructions given to the Candidate

This 13-year-old girl was complaining pain over the back.

What is the finding? Dorsal scoliosis
What are the possible problems associated with this you want to rule out?
Syringomyelia, Tethered cord syndrome, Neurofibromata.

Should you operate on all cases of syringomyelia?
Only if there is a CV junction anomaly.

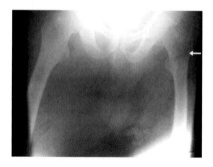

Instructions given to the Candidate

In this poor quality X-ray what do you observe in left hip?
Intertrochanteric fracture.

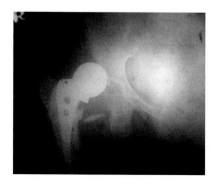

Instructions given to the Candidate

What is the problem here?

Periprosthetic fracture.

Name one classification you know?

Vancouver classification:

A → Inter trochanteric

B → Near the tip

C → Below the tip of the prosthesis

How will you manage?

Traction to bring the head into acetabulum.

Remove the prosthesis and apply longer stem.

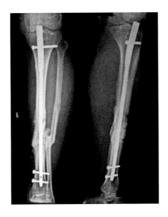

Instructions given to the Candidate

Comment on the implant position?

Nail is longer.

What is the cause?

Availability of the nail.

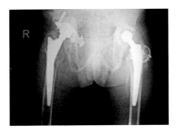

Instructions given to the Candidate

What is seen in the X-ray on acetabular side?

Reconstruction ring on the right side and cemented cupon left side.

What are the possible indications of these implants?

Arthritis of left hip.
Arthritis with protrusion on right side. } Due to rheumatoid arthritis

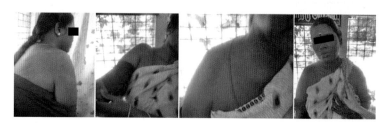

Instructions given to the Candidate

When asked to abduct the shoulder the lady does as shown in Figure 2
What is the diagnosis?
Rotator cuff injury

What will be the other clinical finding?
Wasting of peri-scapular muscles.

How will you investigate?
X-ray of shoulder and neck
MRI cervical spine and shoulder

What are the treatment options available?
Arthroscopic or open repair of the rotator cuff.
Shoot from the screen directly.

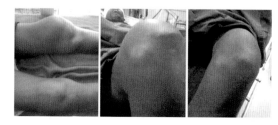

Instructions given to the Candidate

What is the possible diagnosis?
Synovitis of the knee.

What will be the changes in ADL?
Patient cannot squat.

How will you investigate?
X-rays, blood investigations and MRI.

What are the treatment options available?
REST
NSAIDs
Aspiration
Splinting
Specific drugs.

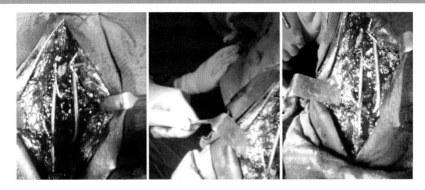

Instructions given to the Candidate

What is the region and what is possibly the fixation?

Spine-region
Luque rod fixation.

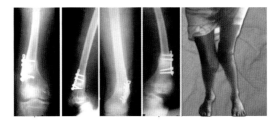

Instructions given to the Candidate

**After a surgery on both knees the patient is seen in the figure.
What is the result?**
Inadequate correction.

Reason for this?
Less wedge taken during the surgery.
Less stronger fixation.

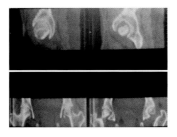

Instructions given to the Candidate

This patient had severe pain in the both hips. He has a childhood history of pain groin and hospitalization.

What is the possible diagnosis this patient had since childhood?
Perthes disease.

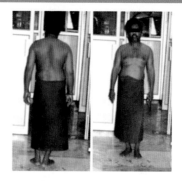

Instructions given to the Candidate

What is the finding?

List to left.

What is the side of lesion in relation to the root?

Axillary type of disc if disc is on right side and shoulder type of disc if on left.

Why it happens?

To avoid irritation of the nerves.

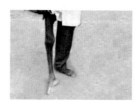

Instructions given to the Candidate

What is this condition?

Residual polio.

What are the usually sparred muscles of lower limb and why?

Peroneus brevis.

Tensor fascia femoris.

They are supplied by more number of roots.

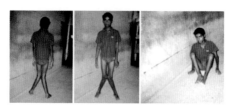

Figures 1 and 2 show patient standing and in figure 3 he is sitting.

What is the diagnosis?

Genu valgus.

In which bone there is the deformity?

Femur.

What will be the changes in ADL and other finding?
Difficulty in walking and squatting.

How will you investigate?
X-ray of both knees AP is standing position.

Name the surgery?
Macewen's osteotomy.

How it will correct the deformity?
A wedge of bone is taken with base facing medially.

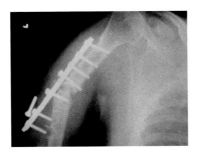

What shall be the reason for this?
Less screws in the distal fragment, screws close to fracture site
Infection of the implant.
Over drilling.
Porotic bone.

How will you treat this condition?
Interlocking nail
Longer broad DCP, locking plate with bone grafting.

What biological method will you prefer?
Dual onlay bone graft.

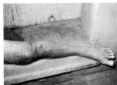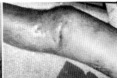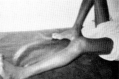

Instructions given to the Candidate

This 40-year-old man had pain and swelling of his left knee. This is the clinical finding.

What are the deformities?
Triple deformity of knee

What is the main diagnosis to be ruled out?
TB Knee

Investigations?
MRI
TB PCR.

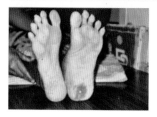

Instructions given to the Candidate

This 45-year-old lady had a draining sinus from the left heel (see above)

What are the clinical findings?
Widened heel
Sinus draining

What are the investigations?
CT scan of the calcaneum.

What is the incision to eradicate infection?
Midline sagittal incision.

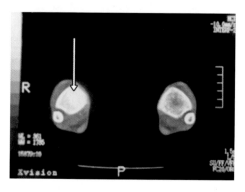

Instructions given to the Candidate

A 29-year-old gentleman came with pain in right lower leg without any external swelling, pain was more during midnight. This is his CT scan.

What is the probable diagnosis?
Osteoid osteoma.

What drug specifically relieves the pain?
Aspirin.

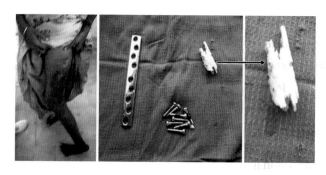

What are the less invasive options you know to treat this condition?
Ablation

Instructions given to the candidate

This patient had a surgery for injury in the thigh 2 years back. Now she is able to walk but had persistent watery discharge from the lower thigh. she underwent surgery for the same.

What is the diagnosis?
Patient with femur osteomyelitis

The second photo shows the things removed during surgery. What are they?
Broad Dynamic Compression Plate, screws and Sequestra are removed

What is the enlarged view of the things removed shown in third photo?
Sequestrum.

How will you identify this 3rd picture if it was given in your hand?
Sequestrum is identified by **Ivory** white colour, **Smooth** side (on the pus), **Rough** side (Granulation side), **Dull** note on dropping down, **sinks** in water whereas a normal bone will float.

What are types of this lesion in adult?
Cierny- Mader type of osteomyelitis in adult.
A. Medullary
B. Superficial cortex
C. Localized cortical and medullary
D. Diffuse cortical and medullary (unstable).

Host classified as:
A - Healthy
BS - Compromise due to Systemic factors
BL - Compromise due to Local factors
BLS -- Compromise due to both Local and Systemic factors
C – Treatment worst than disease

What is the investigation of choice in acute form of this disease?

3 phase bone scan: It differentiate acute osteomyelitis and cellulitis. Former will have activity in delayed images, latter has normal activity in delayed images.

There is a sinus will you do any specific investigation regarding this? What is its importance?

Sinogram. It is better to open the window at the site of the sinus rather than normal bone to not to weaken the cortex in the already diseased bone.

What are the causes of persisting sinus?

1. Non-dependant drainage.
2. Epithelialisation of tract.
3. Low grade infection of tract.
4. Resistant bacteria.
5. Immunocompromised host.
6. Presence of foreign body.
7. Specific infection like TB.

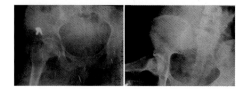

What is this view?

AP and frog lateral views

What are its uses?

This gives an idea of the femoral head and neck in two dimensions.

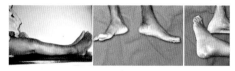

From these pictures what is apparently seen?

Apparent shortening of the right lower limb.

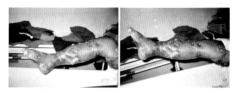

This 40-year-old may had Ilizarov ring removal done 15 days back. He is asked to do certain maneuvers what are they?

The patient is asked to do straight leg rising.

What is the inference?

He is able to do lift the leg and do straight leg rising, so fracture is considered to be united.

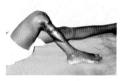

This man had circumferential skin loss in leg following a crush injury. What will be the problem in his lower limb?

Lymphedema.

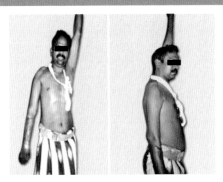

This 40-year-old gentleman was thrown away from a two wheeler.

What is the problem in his right upper limb?

Brachial plexus injury

What are the clinical signs of poor prognosis in this condition?

Involvment of first nerves and all 5 roots; Supraclavicular anesthesia, Pain in an anesthetic limb, Loss of ciliospinal reflex, Horner's syndrome

What ate the findings of poor prognosis in cervical X-ray and Myelogram?

X-ray → Fracture of transverse process

Myelogram → Pseudomeningocele effect.

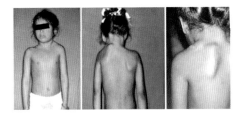

Instructions given to the Candidate

What is the diagnosis of the above child?

Sprengel's shoulder

What are the possible abnormalities you will look for in the X-rays?

Omovertebral bodies

Block vertebra.

What is the treatment of this condition?

Sectioning of scapula longitudinally in the body level. (or)

Releasing the muscles from levator scapula to serratus anterior below.

What will sudden correction of such a deformity will cause?

It can cause neurovascular compromise of the upper limb.

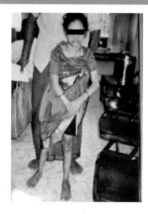

Instructions given to the Candidate

This normally delivered girl had viral encephalitis at 5 years. She is now 11- year old.

What are the tell tale evidences you see on the lower limb of this girl?
Callosities.

What is the possible diagnosis?
Cerebral palsy

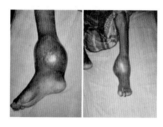

Instructions given to the Candidate

This 17-year-old boy had sudden swelling of his right lower leg with pain. On palpation the swelling was soft vascular mass.

What is the possible clinical diagnosis at this stage?
Malignant bone tumor.

How will the 2 initial imagings you will do?
X-ray of right leg with ankle.
MRI of right leg with ankle.

What will confirm your diagnosis?
Core needle biopsy.

Name 2 investigations to assess the stage of this disease?
CT Chest

Tc 99 scan.

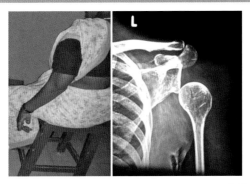

This 40-year-old lady was delivered after a long and difficult lesion and had-deformity since birth. She had inability to flex the elbow, supinate the forearm and flexion of finger abducting the shoulder since childhood

What is the diagnosis?

Erbs palsy.

What is this attitude called?

Waiter's tip receiving position

If it was a child-How will you examine the child 's abilty to move the upper limb? In child -provoking the child to move the upper limb.

What is prognostic indicator?

Biceps within 3 – 6 months after delivery, carries good prognosis.

What are the reconstruction procedures available?

Shoulder arthrodesis in functional position Muscle transfer to augment elbow flexion.

Instructions given to the Candidate

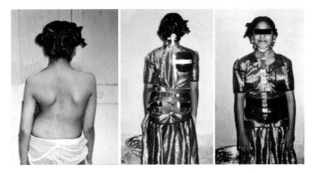

This 10-year-old girl is shown here.
What is her problem?

Dorsal scoliosis with curve on the right side.

Name the appliance on her?

Milwaukee brace.

What is the effect of this appliance on her chin?

Mandibular hypoplasia.

How long will you follow her?

Till skeletal maturity.

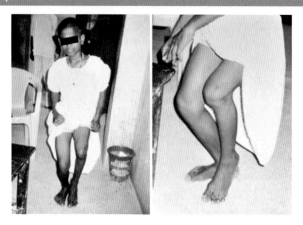

Instructions given to the Candidate

This 15-year-old girl had a difficulty in extending her left knee. She had pain in her knee in her early childhood with history of hospitalisation.

What is her problem?
Subluxed left knee.

How will you investigate?
X-ray. Doppler, MRI.

Name one method to correct this deformity?
Ilizarov.

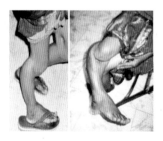

Instructions given to the Candidate

This 18-year-old girl has shortening of her right leg.

What is her problem?
She has gross subluxation of right knee with upper tibia in a posterior relation with lower femur.

How will you investigate?
X-ray, Doppler, MRI.

Name one method to correct this deformity?
Ilizarov.

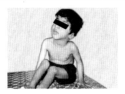

Instructions given to the candidate

This child had been delivered by natural vaginal delivery after prolonged 2nd stage of labor.

What is the cause of this?
Birth anoxia

What is the diagnosis?
Cerebral palsy

Name one question you will ask his mother?
About his first cry.

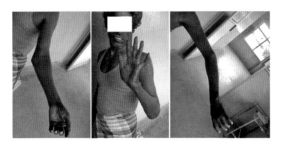

What is this condition?
Cubitus valgus.

Questions on the knowledge of this condition.
What is the 2 important things in the history of this condition?
- History of injury to the elbow.
- History of massage/splinting. (indignous treatment)

Ability to Exam

Greet Explain, get Consent Undresses both upper limbs.
- Compares deformity of valgus if it was more than the normal side. Elicits deformity of elbow in the form of Cubitus valgus
- Feels for Irregularity over lateral condyle of humerus/abnormal mass of the elbow over the lateral condyle.
- Abnormal mobility may or may not be present. Relative mobility to be tested against the humerus.
- Tests for sensation over ulnar nerve area
- Examine for range of movement.

What will you ask the patient to about the feel of his hands?

The patient is asked about numbness of medial one and half fingers and weakness of fingers (intrinsic weakness).

Questions on knowledge of this condition.

What will you expect to see in the X-ray?

Confirm the mal/nonunion

Usually it is difficult to identify the original fracture.

If you have lateral condyle fracture with no abnormal mobility but X-ray shows no Callus. How will you explain ?

Patient is having fibrous union.

Why should this fracture have so common to go for nonunion?

The fracture ends are not opposed to each other. In fact the distal fragment rotates 180 deg and both fracture surfaces are facing laterally.

What is that you see in the same patients hand?

Tardy ulnar nerve palsy

What is the cause of this condition ?

Associated with progressive cubitus valgus due to epiphyseal arrest of the lateral condyle and progressive growth of medical epiphysis. Commonly after epiphyseal injury involving lateral condyle.

What will the patient complain ?

The patient complain numbness of medial one and half fingers and weakness of fingers (intrinsic weakness)

Before attempting any treatment what will you order or do?

Nerve conduction studies.

How will you prevent worsening of this conditiont?

Anterior transposition of ulnar nerve

What is the treatment?

Early cases – anterior transposition of ulnar nerve physiotherapy to the finger. should be decided not later than 3 months of injury.

Later cases – as for ulnar claw hand—tendon transfers

What is cubital tunnel syndrome?

The groove behind the medial epicondyle may be shallow in some individuals. So after a trauma may not be related to this region but a supracondylar fracture etc the patient may experience numbness and weakness of the region of the ulnar nerve.

What is the treatment for this syndrome?

Extension splint –neurovitamins-for a period of 3 months from injury. Nerve conduction studies and the slowing or no conduction confirmed and Anterior transposition of ulnar nerve is done.

What is the complication of this surgery?
Temporary to permanent loss of ulnar nerve function is a known complication

When will you do bony correction?
Osteotomy at second stage, after skeletal maturity
Bone grafting to unite the lateral condyles with minimal fixation

What is the type of osteotomy?
Step cut osteotomy

Why do you need an osteotomy?
To reduce undue loading of medial side of joint.

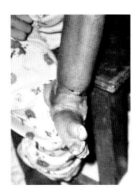

Instructions given to the Candidate

This 25-year-old lady had severe contracture of left ankle following a burns.

What it has produced?
Gross contracture of the medial aspect of ankle, with varus of foot.

How will you correct this?
Ilizarov ring fixator application and gradual correction.

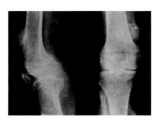

What is the diagnosis?
A neglected fracture of patella.

What will be the clinical sign to test the integrity of this structure?
Active-straight leg raising.

Instructions given to the Candidate

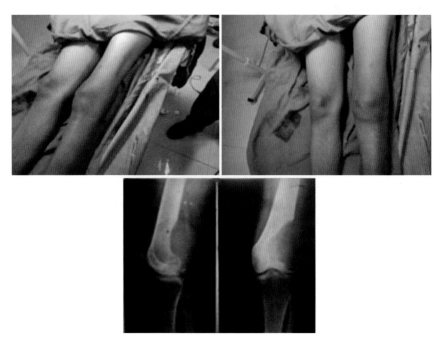

This 30-year-old house wife mother of 2 children came with pain in her left knee for more than three months. She is able to flex her knee but cannot walk.

What is your diagnosis?
Aggressive GCT.

What one investigation you will order?
MRI.

What is the diagnostic test?
Core-Biopsy.

How will you treat this condition?
Resection and reconstruction.

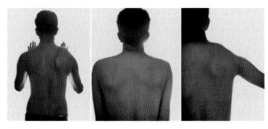

This 19-year-old boy came with difficulty in using his shoulder. He had a viral infection.

On pushing the wall he has prominence of his shoulder blade. Abduction does not reduce prominence.

What is the prominence called?
Winging of scapula

Which muscle will you test?
Serratus anterior muscle.

Test for confirming deltoid fibrosis?
- Abduction must reduce winging.
- Palpate for a band in the deltoid muscle.

No winging on adduction of shoulder, rules out what condition?
Rule out deltoid fibrosis.

Questions on knowledge of this condition.
What are the differential diagnosis of winging of scapula?
1. Weakness of Serratus anterior, due to involvement of long thoracic nerve of Bell.
2. Sprengel's shoulder.
3. Deltoid fibrosis.

Which muscle weakness cause winging?

Serratus anterior holds the medial border of scapula on to the chestwall. So when it is weak, the medial border becomes more prominent or winged– Long thoracic nerve of Bell involvement.

Sprengel's: Scapula is smaller and elevated (Appears to be winged).

Deltoid fibrosis: There is a fixed abduction deformity of the shoulder. So when the arm is brought to the side of chestwall (adduction) scapula appears winged.

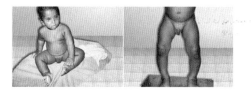

Instructions given to the candidate

In the snaps this 1 ½ year boy has a deformity?
What happened on standing? The deformity is seen.

Where is the deformity?
In femur.

What is the diagnosis? Physiological genu varum.
What are the investigations?
X –ray of both knees to rule out epiphyseal disorders like
Blount's disease, vitamin D level, calcium, phosphorus, ALP.

How will you manage this condition?
Bracing follow up till 3 years, if not corrected spontaneously then intervene.

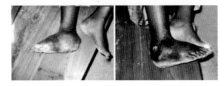

This 45-year-old lady had swelling and multiple sinuses over the foot. She also does not have any pain in the foot or ankle.

What is the diagnosis?
Mycetoma.

What is the associated predisposing condition?
Neuropathy.

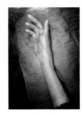

Instructions given to the Candidate

This 35-year-old had severe infection of a finger and had a surgery for that 3 months back.

How many fingers are there?
Four

What is the possible cause?
Amputated index finger for injection (uncontrolld)

You see the limb is draped. What is the possible surgery he may be posted for?
Trimming of the head of 2nd metacarpal.

This 35-year-old man had a fall on the outstretched hand. He has a prominence in the back of the elbow.

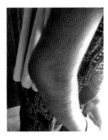

What is the diagnosis?
Unreduced posterior dislocation of elbow.
He demonstrates the triceps standing out (Tendo-Achilles sign of triceps)

Knowledge of this condition
H/o injury, Indigenous treatment usually in splinting extension. restricted movement of elbow.

Fracture disease + over entire upper limb-Skin shiny/Loss of hair +
Triceps standing out (Tendo-Achilles sign of triceps)

What are the treatment options?
Open reduction of the dislocation and mobilization.

Any other procedures to reduce instability?
- Anterior bone block-surgery
- Anterior transposition of triceps
- Ability to exam.
  Looks for ulnar nerve palsy, and 3-point relationship.

What will you tell to educate this patient?
Avoid massaging indigenous splinting for preventing Myositis Ossificans.

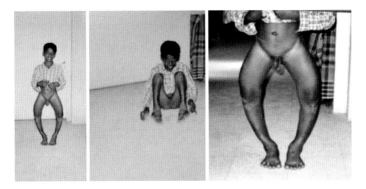

Instructions given to the Candidate

In these snaps, this 12-year-old boy has a deformity?
What happens on sitting in the 2nd photo? Bilateral genu varus disappears
Where is the deformity?
In the femur.

What is the diagnosis?
Genu varum.

What are the investigations?
Standing X-rays of the knee.
Serum calcium phosphorus.
Alkaline-phosphatase.

How will you manage this condition?
Treatment with calcium and vitamin D.
Corrective -osteotomy

What are the treatment options available?

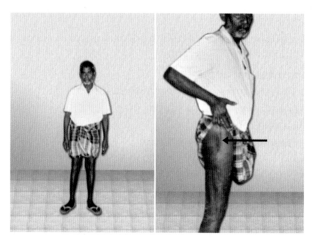

This gentleman shows his scar to you. He had undergone a surgery 1 year back for his pain hip.
He is asked not to squat.
What is the most possible surgery?
Total hip replacement.

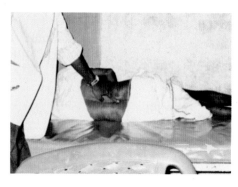

Instructions given to the Candidate

The picture shows a point where this patient has severe tenderness. He also had numbness over left foot and shooting pain over left lower limb

What is the diagnosis?
Intervertebral disc prolapse (Lumbar)

What is the diagnostic investigation?
MRI.

Name one condition that will mimic this diagnosis?
Schwannoma.

What sign can you elicit by pressing on this point?
Tenderness.

What does it mean to have a tenderness?
Instability and inflammation.

Child brought with c/o inability to receive objects (supinate) on the right side. Candidate tests for rotations of the forearm and compares with the neighbor.

Greets the boy. Explains test to him. Gets his consent. Undresses to expose both the upper limbs. Explains the test on the normal side. Asks the patient to do the test on the right side.

O/E :Restricted supination (Rotation),Hypermobility of wrist joint, Forearm fixed in pronation.

Knowledge on the condition?

What is this condition?

Congenital Radio ulnar Synostosis.

What are the types of?

Three types:

1: Upper radius imperfectly formed no head and fused with ulna.

2: Ill formed head of radius attached by a thick interosseous ligament near the coronoid.

3: Head is present malformed –fused with upper ulna.

80% bilateral.

What is the other condition with a similar picture?

Pulled elbow.

What are the treatment options?

Leave alone the child if the child is comfortable. Usually they have hypermobility of the wrist joint and can adjust to all movements except the supination.

If the parents agree to a surgery in spite of thorough explanation—A corrective osteotomy and fixation with forearm in supination

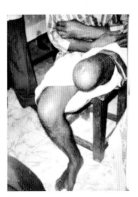

Instructions given to the Candidate

This 30-year-old man had crush injury of his left leg and had a surgery.

What is the present status of his limb?

Thorugh knee stump.

What is your opinion about this stump in view of rehabilitation.?

Bad bulbous stump.

What will you do?
Revision at a higher level.

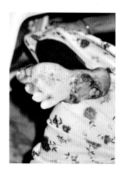

Instructions given to the Candidate

In the photograph you are seeing the foot of a 40-year-old lady.

What is the diagnosis?
Pressure ulcer.

What is the predisposing cause?
Diabetes mellitus.

Name 2 investigations you will order.
Arterial Doppler.
Blood sugar HbA_1C.

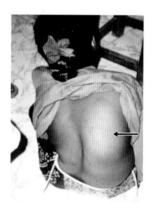

Instructions given to the Candidate

In the photograph you are seeing a lady with deformity of spine.
What is the diagnosis?
Scoliosis.

What are the possible causes?
Idiopathic, polio

What is the prominence on the right side (arrow) is due to?
Rib hump.

What is the cause of it?
Rotation of the dorsal vertebra.

What is the treatment of this hump?

Correcting the scolisosis should correct the hump if not cosmetic – humpectomy can be done by excising the parts of involved ribs.

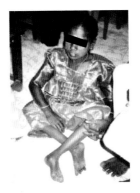

Instructions given to the Candidate

In the photograph you see a lady with weakness of both lower limbs.

What is the diagnosis?

Residual poliomyelitis.

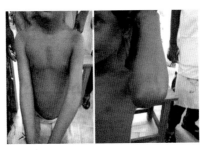

An 8 year old boy is brought with history of fall with injury to the elbow. He had indigenous massage and native splinting. He has difficulty in moving the elbow. What is this deformity? What is the condition?

The gunstock' deformity. Cubitus varus.

What will be the common clinical diagnosis?

Clinically diagnosed as Cubitus varus due to malunited supracondylar fracture with or without myositis ossificans.

Questions on ability

What deformity this patient has.

Cubitus varus

What are the 2 palpatory examinations you will do?

Greet Explain Consent Undresses both upper limbs

- Looks for → Deformity (Gunstock)
- Compares the two supracondylar region of humerus for thickening.
- Looks for ROM – Flexion is restricted usually.

What are the areas to be seen for myositis ossificans?

- Brachialis and triceps.

Questions on the knowledge of this condition.

What is the two important things in the history of this condition?
- History of injury to the elbow.
- History of massage/splinting indigenous treatment.

What is the common reason for which this patient brought to hospital?
Patient usually brought for cosmetic purpose.

What are the investigations and treatment you will order?
X-ray of both elbows – AP – to compare the carrying angle.

What are the treatment options?
Plan: Corrective osteotomy and internal fixation
- French osteotomy
- Step cut osteotomy.

If the patient is in skeletally immature age group, will you not allow for remodelling?
This deformity is in the coronal plane. Remodelling can only occur in the plane of movement of the joint i.e., flexion and extension. In elbow, there is no movement in the coronal plane. Hence remodelling is not possible and hence an osteotomy is a must.

Patient Education.

What shall be your advise if you would have seen this child earlier, immediately after the injury?

Not to massage or to passively move the elbow.

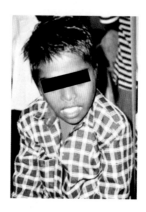

Instructions given to the Candidate

In the photograph you see a boy with a typical facies?

What is it?
Down syndrome.

What are the expected findings in the hands, feet and X-ray pelvis of these children?

Hand: Clinodactyly, single palmar crease–simian crease

Feet: Wide gap between 1st and 2nd toes

X-ray of pelvis: Flat acetabulum and flaring up of iliac wings.

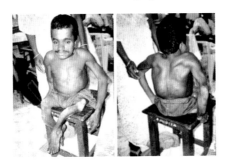

In the photograph you see a man with multiple deformities and typical picture of a problem.

What is the diagnosis?

Osteogenesis imperfecta.

What are the types of the disease?

Sillence classification

4 types.

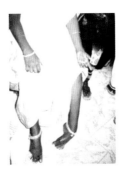

Instructions given to the Candidate

In the photograph you see a lady with a deformity in the foot and ankle.

What is the deformity?

Unilateral neglected clubfoot on the left side.

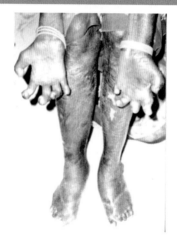

Patient has diminished sensation over both the upper and lower limbs. What is the diagnosis?

Post Hansen sequelae.

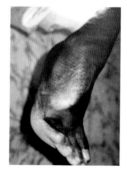

What condition causes this sort of problem?

Neglected clubfoot.

What is the reason to say so?

There is typical deformity with callosity

How will you treat this condition?

Triple arthrodesis.

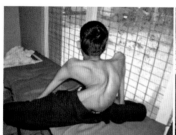
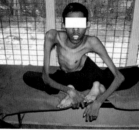
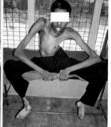

What is the possible cause of this?
Severe poliomyelitis.

Can you correct the spinal deformity now?
Difficult.

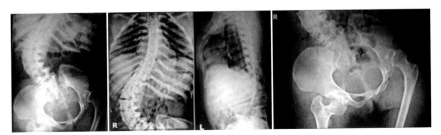

These are X-rays of the above patient
What are the problems in the right hip?
Instability of right hip.

What are the problems of left hip?
Subluxation of left hip.

What are the curves in spine?
Left thoracic and right lumbar curve.

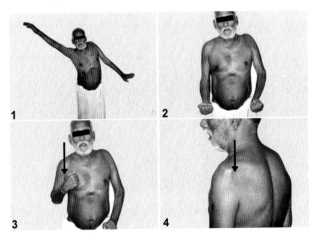

Instructions given to the Candidate

What is that you see in figures 1,2, 3?
Patient tries to abduct his left shoulder, but cannot.

What do you see in figure 4 in the left shoulder region?
Wasting of periscapular muscles.

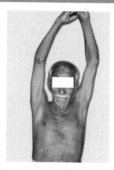

A patient with severe radiating pain in right upper limb. This position relieves his pain.

What is the diagnosis?
Cervical disc prolapse.

What is this sign called?
Relief sign.

What is the diagnostic investigation?
MRI of cervical spine.

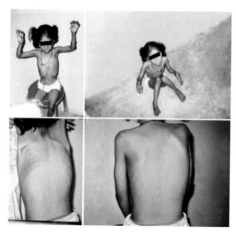

Child is 12-years-old with findings of chest and upper and lower limb deformities.

What is the possible cause?
Rickets.

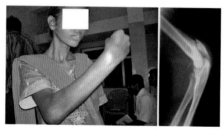

This 20-year-old girl had injury to her right elbow presents after three months with this finding clinically and radilocigally.

What is the condition?

A post-traumatic stiff elbow, myositis ossificans.

What history you need to ask?

H/O injury to elbow and indigenous massage.

What you need to demonstrate?

Demonstrate deformity and range of movement.

Should they always have a bony injury for this condition?
May or may not have bony injury.

What are the common findings?

Range of movement of elbow restricted.
The bony prominences like lateral supracondylar ridge, lateral condyle, radial head, olecranon, medial epicondyle, medial supracondylar ridge in that order is palpated for any irregularity.

What are the treatment options?

Conservative treatment
Indomethacin
Low dose radiation
Active mobilization.

If no improvement-with this conservative treatment what is your plan?

Adhesiolysis/arthrolysis.

What is the minimum requirement of flexion of the elbow joint?

Flexion of the elbow joint should be enough to reach the mouth for the right side.

A 30-year-old has pain and swelling of left elbow.

There is no history of any injury.

There was no H/O fever/morning stiffness.

Questions on ability to exam

In this case where will you look for synovial swelling? What are the bony points you will palpate?

Tenderness and diffuse swelling on either side of olecranon.

Tenderness over Radial head, Lateral Condyle.

Questions on Knowledge. What else will you examine?

To see axillary and supraclavicular nodes.

To see other joint movements.

What is your clinical diagnosis ?

TB/RA

How will you proceed?

Investigation for above two diseases. The X-ray and blood investigation.

What are the treatment options?

Synovectomy or Excision elbow and ATT – For TB.
Synovectomy and Anti-rheumatoid drugs and joint replacement – For RA
Arthroplasty for heated TB and RA.

In which condition of elbow joint replacement is contraindicated ?
Main contraindication is active infection.

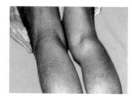

Instructions given to the Candidate

What do you see in the right popliteal fossa, the patient is lying prone?
A popliteal cyst.

What will be the acute presentation of this condition?
Rupture of the sac of the popliteal cyst

How will you treat such condition in a child, a rheumatoid patient and in suspected DVT?

A child → leave alone and observe.

A rheumatoid patient → synovectomy.

In suspected DVT → which may mimic ruptured sac-start the anti-clotting treatment like heparin. Do an ultrasound to find the intactness of the sac, and a doppler to look for DVT.

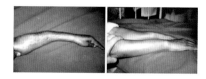

Instructions given to the Candidate

This is the forearm of a 40 year old male who had a fall and indigenous bone setting.

What one clinical examination you will do?
Test for abnormal mobility.

What one movement that will be restricted?
Rotations.

What is the treatment of this condition?
Osteotomy, Realignment and Internal fixation

After 3 months of an injury to left elbow an 8-year-old boy complain numbness of medial one and half fingers and weakness of fingers. What will you look for in this patient?

Look for any irregularity of medial epicondyle.

Carefully look for any involvement of ulnar nerve.

What is this condition?
Medial condyle fracture.

What initial imaging investigations you will order?

X-ray of the elbow.

What are the treatment options?

Non union – small fragment – Excision.

Large fragment - fixation with bone grafting

Before attempting any treatment what will you order or do?

Nerve conduction studies.

What is the treatment?

Early cases – wait for 3 months treating with conservative methods anterior transposition of ulnar nerve physiotherapy to the finger. Should be decided not later than 3 months of injury.

Later cases – as for ulnar claw hand—tendon transfers.

What is cubital- tunnel syndrome?

The groove behind the medial epicondyle may be shallow in some individuals. So after a trauma may not be related to this region but a supracondylar fracture, etc. The patient may experience numbness and weakness of the region of the ulnar nerve.

What is the treatment for this syndrome?

Extension splint –neuro-vitamins-for a period of 3 months from injury. If in this time, nerve conduction studies show slowing or no conduction, anterior transposition of ulnar nerve is done.

What is the complication of this surgery?

Temporary to permanent loss of ulnar nerve function is a known complication.

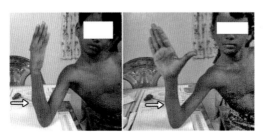

This patient had an injury to his right forearm and was treated conservatively for 4 months.

What is the movement the patient is asked to do?

What movement is restricted?

Supination.

What is the pointed area? What is it due to?

A small prominence or angulation.

A fracture.

What is the diagnosis?

Malunion of both bones of forearm.

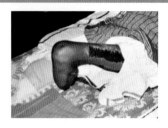

Instructions given to the Candidate

What is the possible cause of that scar on the thigh?
It appears as a donor site for skin grafting.

What is the actual condition of the lower limb?
Below knee amputation.

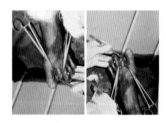

Instructions given to the Candidate

What is the possible procedure?
Shortening closure.

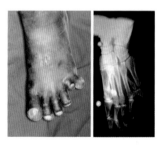

Instructions given to the Candidate

This is a 16-year-old dwarf girl's foot.
What is this condition?
Polydactyly.

What are the associated conditions with this?
Chondrodysplastic dwarfism.
Nail hypoplasia
Narrow acetabulum
Low vaginal atresia.

What is the syndrome associated with dwarfism and polydactyly?
Ellis Van Creveld syndrome.

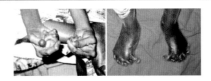

Instructions given to the Candidate

This is a 50-year-old lady's hands and feet.

What is this condition?
Rheumatoid arthritis.

What are the types of joint involvement in this?
Small joints of the hand and feet like MCP, MTP, IP joints.

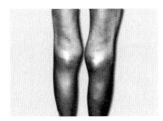

Instructions given to the Candidate

This is a 50-year-old gentleman who had severe pain in both knees. His both knees are seen from behind.
What is this condition?
Bilateral popliteal cysts.

What is the usual associated condition with this?
Osteo arthritis of knee joints.

How will you manage this?
Treatment of primary osteoarthritis.
Excision only if it is not resolved with this.

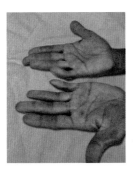

This 45-year-old carpenter an epileptic patient on drugs who used to work on with vibratory instruments has this finding in his both hands. What is the condition? What is the possible pathology?

Dupuytren's contracture.

Fibrosis and contracture of MCP joint. Thickening of palmar fascia – little and ring fingers.

How will you look for the affected structure?

Feel for nodularity of affected finger.

Fibrous strand cross the crease into the affected finger.

How will you differentiate this from claw hand?

There is hyperextension of MCP joint in claw hand but only flexion contracture of IP joints in Dupuytren 's contracture.

Candidate is expected to do the following:

He - Greets –Explains test –gets consent- Undresses adequately. palpates for nodularity of the affected finger along the palmar aponeurosis strips other fingers and contralateral side.

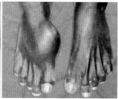

Instructions given to the Candidate

This 30-year-old lady presented with a firm swelling over the dorsum of foot. There is restricted movement of the great toe.

What is the probable diagnosis?

GCT of the tendon sheath.

What investigation you order to diagnose this condition?

MRI of the foot.

How will you treat this condition?

Excision of the tumor.

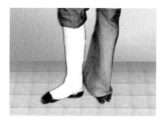

Instructions given to the Candidate

What type of plaster of Paris cast is this?

This is a special cast called MNOH cast which is a modification of the PTB.

The foot touches the ground directly (MN Orthopedic Hospital-Cast).

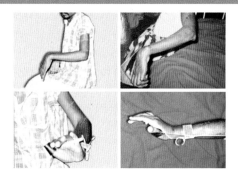

Instructions given to the Candidate

What is the diagnosis?
Wrist and finger drop.

What is the possible cause, from the figure?
Direct cut of the nerve by an assault.

What is the splint given?
Dynamic wrist drop splint.

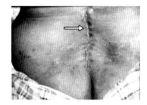

Instructions given to the Candidate

What is seen in the picture of back of a person?
Scar of a spinal surgery.

What are the possible interventions that would have caused?
Discectomy
Spinal fusion
Spinal trauma instrumentation.

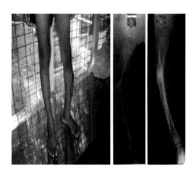

This 8-year-old boy was brought for a deformity of the leg in the form of anterior bowing from birth.

He had a history of indigenous treatment.

How will you examine him pertaining to this deformity?

Candidate should

- Look for deformity – the plane – anterolateral
- Look for abnormal mobility m/3 of leg
- Look for neurocutaneous markers

What are the types of this lesion?

BOYD classification

6 types

- 1-Defect
- 2-Hourglass
- 3-Cyst
- 4-Sclerosis
- 5-Dysplasia of fibula
- 6-Interosseous fibroma.

Name one consistent finding in all types. What will you see in the X-ray?

Thickening of fibula and thinning of the tibial shaft.

What are surgical options?

Ideally resection of the pseudoarthrosis and bone transport with Ilizarov.

The other options are vascularized fibular graft, bone grafting and internal fixation.

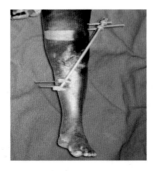

Instructions given to the Candidate

What is this ?

Knee spanning fixator.

What are the possible indication of this ?

Temporary stabilization of intra articular fractures of proximal tibia or distal femur.

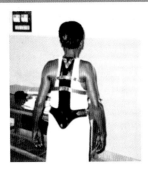

Instructions given to the Candidate

Name the appliance?
Taylor's brace

What is the technical name for this?
TLSO (Thoraco Lumbo Sacral Orthosis).

What is the possible indication?
Dorsal spine injury.

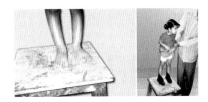

Instructions given to the Candidate

**This child was treated with serial plasters from birth
This is the present condition.
What is the possible condition?**
Congenital Talipes Equino Varus (corrected).

What is the appliance given?
Clubfoot boot.

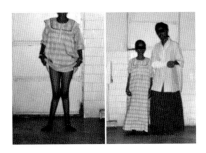

Instructions given to the Candidate

**The lady in the 1st frame is seen with her younger sister in the next figure.
What is the possible diagnosis?**
Renal rickets.

What one imaging apart from knee X-rays you will order and why?
Ultrasound of abdomen to find kidney size and corticomedullary differentiation.

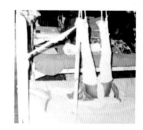

Instructions given to the Candidate
What is this ?
Gallow's traction

What is the indication?
Fracture shaft of femur- unilateral or bilateral

In what age group this is advocated?
2-4 years of age group

What is the complication of this procedure?
Avascular necrosis of femoral head.

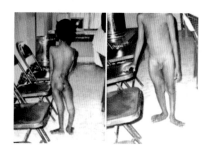

This boy was operated for a congenital spinal condition.
He has weakness of both lower limbs and incontinence of bladder.

Name the condition.
Spina bifida.

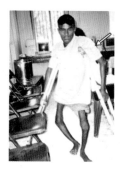

Instructions given to the Candidate

What does this boy has?

This boy had bilateral residual poliomyelitis

What will be the complication he will develop on his left side upper limb?

Klumpke's palsy.

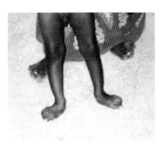

What is this condition?

Severe flat feet.

What one codition you will rule out?

Congenital vertical talus.

What is the special foot wear?

Robert Jones- C & E heel, Crooked and Elongated heel.

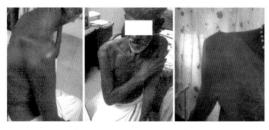

This 50-year-old man fell on an outstretched hand and had loss of movements of his right shoulder immediately. Look if the candidate asks the patient to sit with both shoulders bare

Name 2 inspectory findings in this case seen from front of the patient (figure 3)?.

Loss of contour of shoulder.

Anterior axillary fold is at lower level (Bryant's sign)

Name three tests

Please see if the candidate keeps a ruler on lateral condyle of the affected side humerus and finds if it touches the affected side acromion (Hamilton ruler test positive) or not. It usually donot touch because of resistance of head. In dislocated case, the ruler touches the acromion.

Please see if the candidate asks the patient to touch the opposite shoulder (Dugas test) the patient cannot.

Please see if the candidate measures the vertical circumference at both the axillae are increased (Callaway sign)

What are the treatment options in this patient?
Depends on age.
As this patient is in between age, Open reduction if patient is young, Mobilize if old patient.

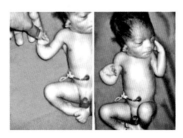

What is this condition?
Radial club hand.
This extreme radial deviation of wrist, fingers touching the forearm.

What will the X-ray possibly show?
Partial or complete absence of the radius.

What are the associated conditions?
Thrombocytopenia
Absent Radius,
Tetralogy of Fallot's
Atrial septal defect.

What is the treatment of this case?
Initial splinting of the forearm.
Later excision of the lunate and fusion of the wrist with centralization of the ulna.

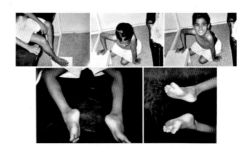

Instructions given to the Candidate

This 10-year old boy can sit on the chair as in first figures.
But when he was asked to get up from floor. See what happens in figures 2 and 3.
He is not able to get up from the floor on his own.
The fourth figure shows his calf. What is this called?
Pseudo hypertrophy of calf.

What does the 5th figure show?
Bilateral equines.

What is your diagnosis?
Duchenne muscular dystrophy.

What are the systems this affects?
Cardiac muscles

What are the lab tests you will order?
Creatinine-phosphokinase level

What is the diagnostic test?
Muscle biopsy.

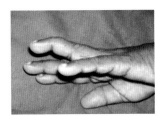

What is this condition?
Mallet finger.

What is the pathology?
Characterized by flexion of DIP joint due to avulsion of long extensors from the distal insertion/Passive extension is possible in early cases.

What would be the X-ray picture?
Avulsion of distal phalanx.

What is the treatment?
Volar splinting in IP extension – 6 weeks.
Repair and suturing by a transverse elliptical incision .

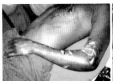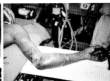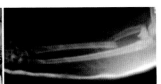

Instructions given to the Candidate

This 22-year-old man had a left forearm injury in a vehicular accident. These are his clinical pictures and X-ray.

What are his injuries in the forearm?
Fracture shaft of radius and its neck.

How will you manage them?
Being in adult excision of radial head and fixation of the shaft fracture; Grafting the fracture with the excised head of radius.

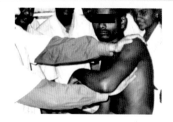

Instructions given to the candidate.

What is this examination aimed at?
To palpate the axillary lymph nodes.

In orthopedics what is the need for such an examination?
In case of infection or tumors of soft tissue of the upper limb it is necessary to examine the axillary lymph nodes.

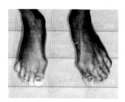

Instructions given to the Candidate

What is this condition?
Rheumatoid feet-Hallux valgus.
Name one recent injectable immumological drug?
Etaner

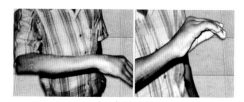

Instructions given to the Candidate

This 25-year-old male had a forearm surgery done 6 weeks back. (see the scar).
He is asked to do dorsiflexion.

O/E this was the inspection- finding of little finger

What is the problem in this patient?
Claw hand.

What is the test you will do to find the structure weakened by this causing the deformity?
Power of the intrinsic muscles

What is the structure which can be substituted the above weakness?

Flexor digitorum superficialis (FDS)

What is the name of the splint you will prescribe?

Knuckle-bender splint.

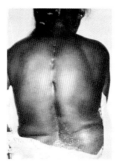

This is a case of spinal deformity operated when she was 12-year-old. Now at 40 years she has pain in the upper back.

What is the possible surgery done ?

Scoliosis correction.

What is the cause of the present problem?

Implant cut through due to osteoporosis.

Implant loosening due to skeletal growth.

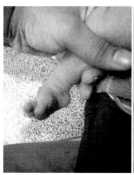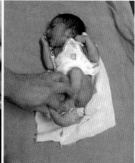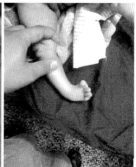

This is a picture of a newborn. The next two pictures during the course of treatment.

What is the condition?

Congenital talipes equinovarus.

What is the technique?

Ponsetti casting technique.

What are the steps of treatment completed, what are left?

The cavus is corrected.

Adduction, Varus, Equines are left.

A 50-year-old non diabetic lady had a wrist injury on her right side and had indigenous massage and splinting. After 4 months she has severe burning sensation and pain all over the right upper limb which did not confine to wrist.

What is her condition called?

RSD.

How will you classify this condition?

RSD is a group of conditions occurring after trauma classified into minor causalgia, major causalgia, minor traumatic dystrophy, major traumatic dystrophy, shoulder hand syndrome.

What are the stages of this disease?

Stage 1 : Burning aching pain.
Stage 2 : Edema, Cold glossy skin and joint stiffness.
Stage 3: Progressive atrophy of skin and muscle and significant joint contracture.

Why her pain not localized?

Short circuiting of nerves is proposed, and hence the pain is non-anatomic.

What are the treatment options?

Initially physiotherapy, Calcium ,Calcitonin can be tried along with analgesics. Later on Sympathetic block. Progressive loading of extremity and progressive resistant exercises.

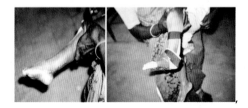

Instructions given to the Candidate

What is the probable surgery done?
Posteromedial release for clubfoot

How will you say so?
Scar of the incision is at posteromedial site.

What is the name of the splint?
Below knee splint.

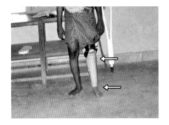

Instructions given to the Candidate

What is this prosthesis?
Patellar tendon bearing prosthesis.

What is the indication of this prosthesis?
Below knee amputation.

What is special about the part marked below?
SACH (Solid Ankle Cushion-Heel).

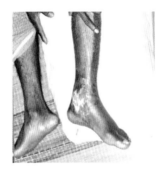

Instructions given to the Candidate

**This is a non-healing ulcer following an injury of the ankle.
What two investigations you will order: One—imaging
and One—blood investigation?**
Venous Doppler and GTT.

Chapter 3

Model OSCE Problems Part 2

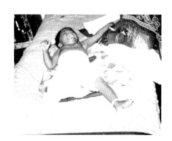

Instructions given to the Candidate

What is this plaster?

1 ½ hip spica.

What is the region that can be immobilized with this?

Upper femur injury like
- Neck of femur fractures
- Trochanteric fractures, and femoral shaft fractures

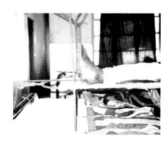

Instructions given to the Candidate

What is this appliance?

BB Splint or Bohler–Braun splint.

How will you select the length of this splint?

It has a limb rest with a genu corresponding to the knee.

What is the procedure done here?

The limb is kept in BB splint with calcaneal pin traction.

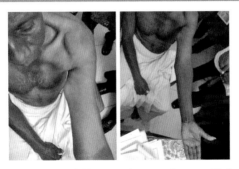

This 45-year-old man had diffuse pain on the medial two fingers and the adjoining part of hand and distal medial forearm. He also has a swelling on the medial side of the arm which moves side-to-side and not longitudinally. There is no specific deformity of fingers.

What is the possible diagnosis of this swelling?

Nerve sheath tumour of ulnar nerve.

Why it has caused this finding?

There is possibly pressure on sensory fibers only.

Why there is no specific deformity of fingers?

Since the ulnar nerve lesion is high there may not be prominent clawing.

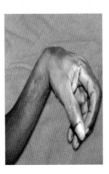

This boy had sudden deformity after a surgery over arm. He also had numbness over the dorsum of hand.

What is the diagnosis?

Postoperative wrist drop.

What are the components of the affected structure?

Sensory and motor.

Ability

→ **Checks the autonomous region of sensory supply of this nerve.**

GECU

Exposes entire upper limbs.

Explains test in the normal limb.

Asks the patient to tell 'one' or 'yes ' if he feels the sensation of touch.

Tests the sensation of the affected side.

Tests for anesthesia present over 1st web space over the dorsal aspect and compares with the other.
Palpates the entire course of radial nerve to look for tenderness
(Radial nerve ends at the level of lateral condyle and continues as Posterior Interosseous nerve to midpoint of wrist).
Motor
Power of wrist extensor and finger and thumb extensor.

What is the treatment of this condition?

Initial – Splinting in volar cock-up splint, Nerve conduction tests if the recovery is not there, then tendon transfer

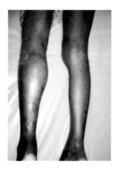

Instructions given to the Candidate

This 45-year-old smoker had severe swelling of left calf?
What are the differential diagnosis?

Deep vein thrombosis, thrombo angitis obliterans

How will you investigate?

Arterial and venous Doppler.
D-dimer ultrasound scan of popliteal region to look for intactness of the popliteal sac.

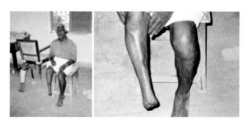

Instructions given to the Candidate

What is done to the right lower limb?

Syme's amputation.

Name two other similar procedures at this level.
Pirogoff's amputation
Chopart's amputation.

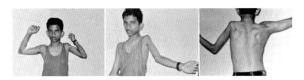

Instructions given to the Candidate

This 14-year-old boy came with this finding, what is the diagnosis. What he able to do in the first snap?
Flex both the elbows.

What is he is trying to do in the second snap?
Abducting the left shoulder **The undressed view of the same attempt seen from behind. What he is trying to do?**
Abducting the shoulder.

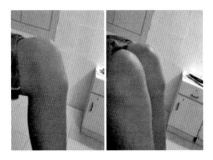

Instructions given to the Candidate

These are the clinical pictures of an adolescent boy who had pain over the tibial tuberosity. How will you examine?

In Manned Station
Look for swelling, prominence and tenderness over the tibial tuberosity. Look for range of movement.

Flexion almost full except mild restriction in the extreme flexion.

In Unmanned Station
1. **What is the diagnosis?**
2. **What will you see in the X-ray?**
3. **What is the treatment?**

Answers
1. Osgood Schlatter's disease
2. Fragmentation of the tibial tuberosity apophysis.
3a. Extension splints, NSAIDs
3b. Excision of the fragment.

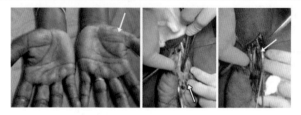

Instructions given to the Candidate

This 40-year-old lady had pain and numbness in her hand and outer fingers of her left hand.

What is the arrow pointing in the 1st picture?
Thenar muscle wasting in the left side.

What is the arrow pointing in the 2nd picture? What is released?
The flexor retinaculum is being released.

What structure is being released as the arrow pointing in the 3rd picture?
Median nerve.

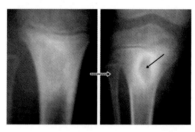

An 8-year-old girl was brought for pain in her knee joint after a dance program in her school.

The first picture showed her initial X-ray. She was diagnosed and was put on specific medication. The result was pain relief and the fresh X-ray revealed in the second picture.

What was possible diagnosis?
TB osteomyelitis.

What was the possible medication?
Anti-tuberculous medication.

In follow-ups of the child how will you assess the activity of the disease?
Periodic ESR.

What is the finding in the second X-ray that shows healing of the disease?
Sclerosis.

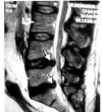 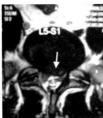 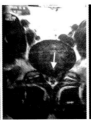 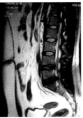

Instructions given to the Candidate

From the first MRI picture even without an X-ray LS spine lateral view can you tell if there will be sacralization or not?
There cannot be sacralization.

Why?
If so, then L5 S1 disc will be rudimentary and L5 S1 disc would have not prolapsed.

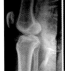 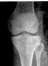 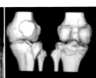 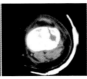 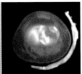

Instructions given to the Candidate

What is the diagnosis?
Split fracture of the lateral condyle.

How will you manage it?
Percutaneous cannulated cancellous screw fixation of the fracture.

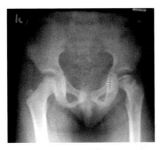

Pain in the left hip since 6 months. Patient is having a persistent limp.
What is the diagnosis?
Perthe's disease.

What is the prognosis?
The entire head is involved, hence poor prognosis.

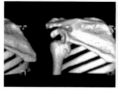 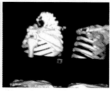

Instructions given to the Candidate

The above is the reconstruction CT of a left shoulder of a 70-year-old post-menopausal lady who had a fall 7 months back.
What is the diagnosis?
Neglected dislocation of left shoulder.

How will you manage her?
Accept the dislocation and mobilize her.

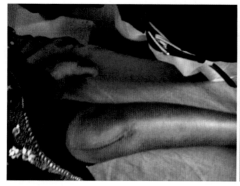 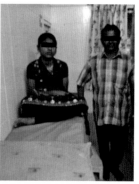

What is the scar?
Scar of an anteromedial incision.

What are the possible surgeries with this incision?
Fixation of intraarticular fragments, e.g. Tibial spine avulsion, synovectomy, arthrolysis.

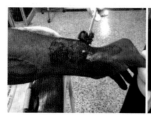 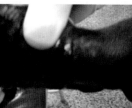 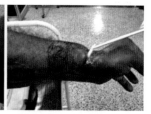

A 40-year old presented with a draining sinus.
What is being done in these steps in figures 1, 2 and 3?
1. The sinus site is swabbed with antiseptic to prevent contamination
2. The sinus is milked.
3. The swab is placed in the site of the sinus to take the swab.

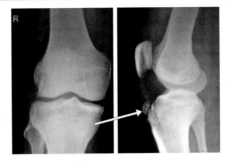

What is the possible diagnosis?

Calcification of ligamentum patella near the Tibial tuberosity.

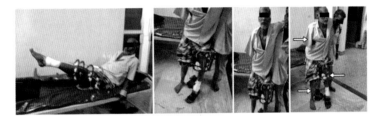

This man has lost right arm below the shoulder level and lost his right thigh above the knee level.

He also had a fractured left distal femur

How is the patient made to raise and walk? What are pointed with the brown blue and black arrows?

His left lower limb fracture was treated with Ilizarov fixation. (left side arrow)

He was given an artificial limb (right lower arrow) for his right amputated stump.

He was made to weight bear with a support of a person.

Right upper arrow shows the amputated right upper limb.

Kumaravel S. Technique of Treating Fractures in Long Bones of Lower Limb with Associated Simultaneous Loss of Limbs in the Same Injury Complicating Their Treatment. Res J Pharmaceut Biol Chem Sci. 2015 6(4): 558-62.

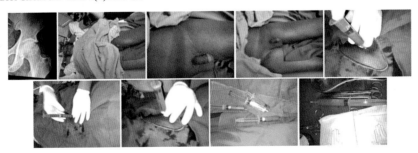

This is a 45-year-old patient with renal failure. He had pain over left groin and fever. What is the procedure being done?

Hip aspiration.

What is the landmark for the procedure?

Femoral pulse is palpated and the needle is put perpendicular to the skin, lateral to the pulsation.

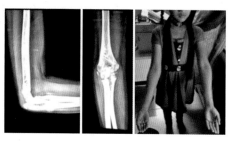

Is there a deformity in the left elbow? Is there a valgus? See the X-ray also before answering?

The forearm appears in line with the arm.

There is no valgus.

How can this elbow be called?

Cubitus rectus.

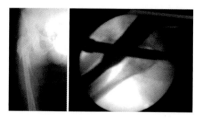

What is the fracture and the C-arm picture shown near?

Proximal femur fracture.

Proximal femoral nailing with zig.

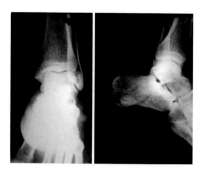

What is the fracture?

Calcaneal fracture.

What is the problem here?

Intra-articular fracture.

What is the difficulty in treating this fracture operatively?

It is difficult to fix these fractures.

What is the long-term result of a malunion of this fracture?

Subtalar arthritis

Peroneal tendon irritation.

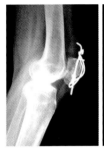 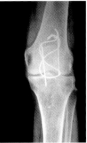

When will you mobilize the knee after this surgery?

Immediately after surgery

When it will affect the apposition of the fracture?

No, it will only compress the fracture.

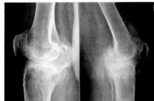 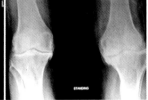

What is the possible condition?

Osteoarthritis of the both knees

What is the option if pain is unbearable with conservation like drugs and physiotherapy?

Total knee replacement.

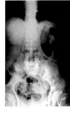 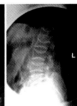 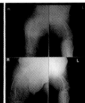 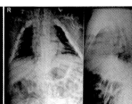

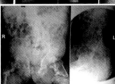

This 60-year-old gentleman had repeated fractures and came for deformity of the lower limb. He was brought in a wheelchair.

With pain right thigh on 20-1-2011. He is a known patient of a childhood disease. Earlier in 1990 he had a hip fracture and in 1998 he had a stroke. One year later he had a fall and had a left thigh fracture. He also has increased renal parameters now.

He has right femur fracture and left distal femur fracture. What is the diagnosis?

Osteogenesis imperfecta.

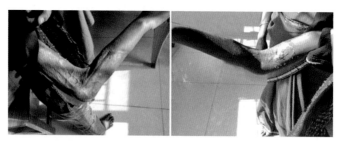

These are is a clinical pictures of a 20-year-old boy.

He had a surgery done 7 years back for a crush injury of the upper limb. In the 1st picture he is asked to flex the elbow and in the 2nd he is asked to extend.

What is the surgery?

Split thickness skin grafting for crush injury and raw area

What is your diagnosis after seeing these movements?

Post-traumatic stiffness of elbow joint.

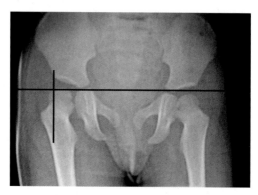

What are these lines?

Vertical lines are Perkin's lines and Horizontal lines are Hilgenreiner's lines.

What is your inference after seeing the lines?

The hip is in situ.

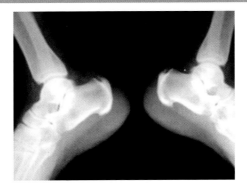

What is the view?
Lateral view of both the heels.

What are the two common indications of this view?
Retro calcaneal bursitis, plantar fasciitis.

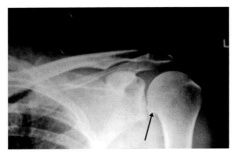

In the glenohumeral joint what is pointed? Is it coomon to see this here?
An osteophyte.
No, it is not common.

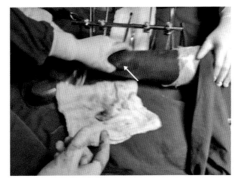

This 30-year-old trauma victim had an external fixation done 1 month back. He was taken for a surgery to improve his chances of union. The incision pointed is on the lateral side. A material which was harvested is seen on a pad.

What is this surgery?

Posterolateral bone grafting.

What are the pre-requisites of this surgery?

An intact fibula

A fracture of the lower third tibia.

Is infection of the fracture a contraindication of this procedure?

No. Actually it is recommended in infected nonunions.

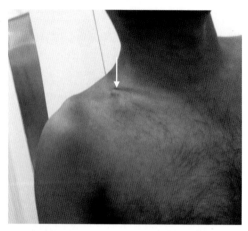

A 30 year old fell from his bike two weeks back. What is the lesion?

Fracture clavicle with end of the proximal fragment tenting the skin.

What are the investigations to confirm the diagnosis?

Radiograph of the shoulder with entire clavicle.

What treatment would you recommend?

Open reduction and internal fixation.

Is there a way you can maintain the length of the bone during above procedure?

An umbilical tape can be used to measure the normal side clavicle and autoclaved and used to reconstruct the injured clavicle.

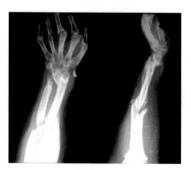

What are the problems of this forearm?

Cross union, Deformity, Osteoporosis.

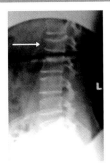

This 45-year-old man had a fall in his work place and landed on his heel. He had pain back. He did not have lower limb weakness or numbness. He passed urine voluntarily after the fall.

What is the diagnosis?

Wedge compression fracture of L1 vertebra.

What is the classification of this injury?

Type 1 Danis classification.

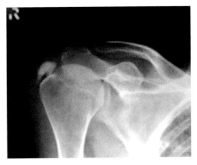

This 40-year-old lady had pain in the right shoulder. This is her X-ray.

What is her diagnosis?

Calcification of supraspinatus tendon.

How will you treat her?

Aspiration of the calcific deposit and injection of hydrocortisone.

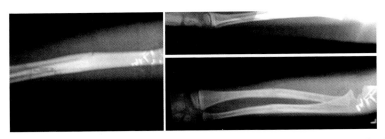

This 7-year-old boy had a fall in school and came with pain in the left upper limb. What is this condition?

Greenstick fracture.

Shall we leave him alone?

We have to correct the deformity and apply plaster.

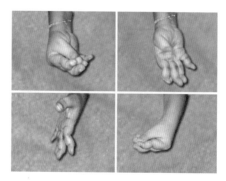

What is the diagnosis?

Rheumatoid hand

Name the predominant deformity in all the fingers?

Swan neck deformity.

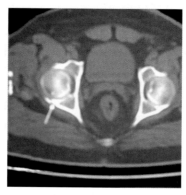

What is the investigation?

CT scan of pelvis.

What is the region?

Hip joint.

What is seen?

A letabular rim fracture-right side

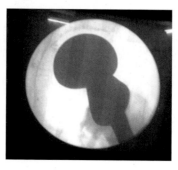

What possibly is this investigation? What is the possible indication?
C-arm picture of an hemiarthroplasty done for fracture Neck of Femur to check reduction.

What is the implant used?
Bipolar hemiarthroplasty

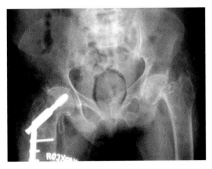

What is your inference on right side and left side?
DHS done for old interochanteric fracture right side
Unoperated neck of femur fracture left side.

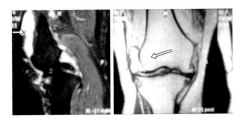

This 40-year-old lady had non-traumatic effusion of her knee. In the MRI what is pointed?
Synovial effusion.

What are the serological tests you will order?
TB ELISA
TB PCR
RA Factor.

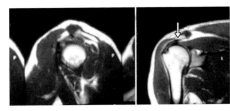

This 37-year-old male had severe pain after a fall with difficulty in active abduction.

This was his MRI. What is the pointed structure?
Supraspinatus tendon.

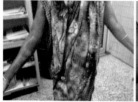 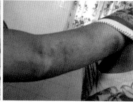

What is this?

Ecchymosis.

What will be the associated hematological finding in this patient?

Anemia.

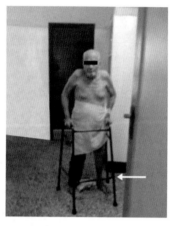

What is the pointed structure?

A walker.

What else you see in this figure?

A knee brace.

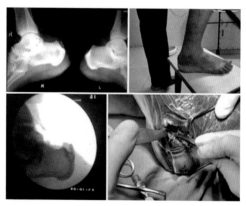

What is the condition seen in pictures 1 and 2?

Retrocalcaneal bursitis.

What is the deformity called?
Haglund-deformity.

What is the surgery done for this?
Excision of the posterior tuberosity of calcaneum.

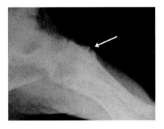

What is the pointed lesion?
Cuneiform metatarsal arthritis.

What shall be the presenting complaint of the patient?
Pain on standing for a long duration.

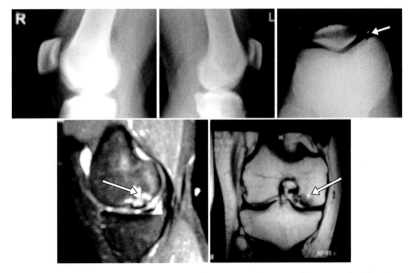

This 20-year-old adolescent boy had a vehicular accident. He had pain on climbing stairs and swelling of the knee.
What do you see in the X-rays?
Osteochondral fracture.

What do you see in the MRI?
Osteochondral fracture.

How best you can treat this condition?
By arthroscopy.

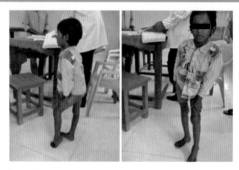

What is the muscle affected in this side?
Quadriceps

What are the associated problems seen?
Tendo-Achilles contracture.

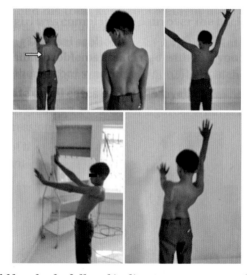

**This 14-year-old boy had a fall and indigenous massage to his left shoulder
What is that he is asked to do?**
He is asked to push against the wall.

What is the observation you see?
The scapula becomes more prominent.

What is your inference?
There is weakness of the serratus anterior muscle.

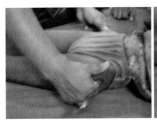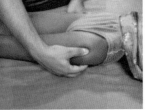

What is being done?
Palpating the greater trochanter levels.

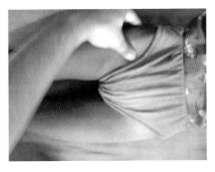

What is being done?
Palpating the greater trochanter for tenderness and thickening (bimanual palpation).

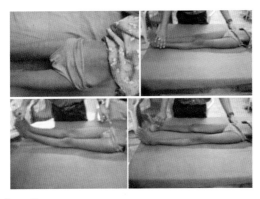

What is being done?
Squaring the pelvis.

What is pointed by the examiner?
The anterior superior iliac spine.

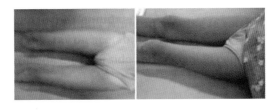

What is shown?
Wasting of left thige muscles.

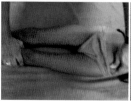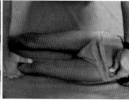

What is being done?
Rotations tested for left hip.

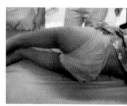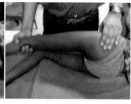

What is being done?
Patient is turned to see the gluteal region.

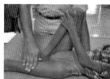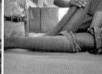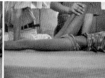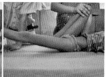

What is being done?
Thomas hip knee flexion test.

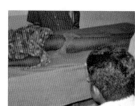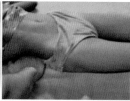

The patient is being inspected from the sides. What is being observed?
The lumbar lordosis is observed if it was exaggerated.

In the next picture what is being done?
Exaggerated lumbar lordosis is palpated.

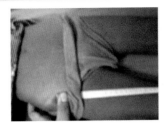

What is being done?
The measuring tape is kept at ASIS for measurement.

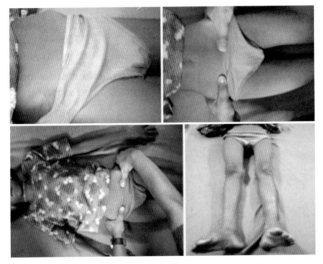

The patient is being inspected, what is being observed in 1st figure?
The ASIS are seen.

In the next 2 pictures, what is being done?
Level of ASIS is palpated.

What is seen in last figure?
Attitude of both the lower limbs is seen.

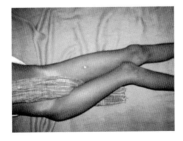

What is seen?
The attiiude of the lower limb.

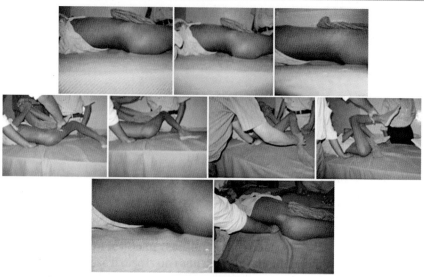

What is being done?

The lumbar lordosis is palpated and Thomas hip knee flexion test is done.

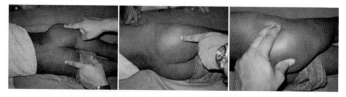

What is being shown in figure 1?

The two gluteal regions are compared.

What is being shown in figure 2?

Prominence in the right gluteal region.

What is being done in figure 3?

The gluteal mass is palpated and femur is rotated to find whether the mass is continuous with femur.

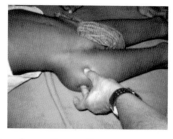

What is being shown in above figure ?

Greater trochanter is palpated.

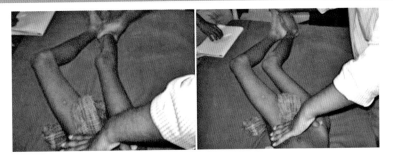

What is being shown in above figure ?
ASIS held by one hand and squaring is done

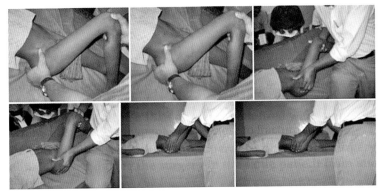

What is being shown in above figures?
Abnormal mobility in the form of telescopy is tested in the right hip.

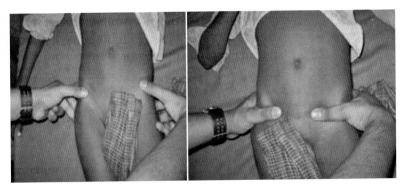

What is being shown in above figures?
Level of ASIS is palpated and compared.

What is the inference?
Right ASIS is at a higher level.

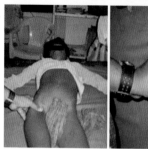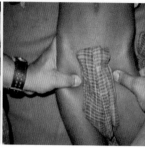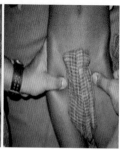

What is being shown in figures?
Femoral artery is palpated both the sides.

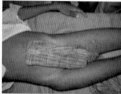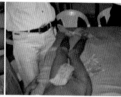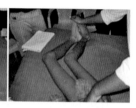

What is being done?
The pelvis is squared.

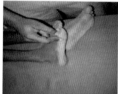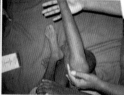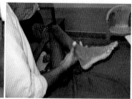

What is being shown in figures?
Checking for hip rotations.

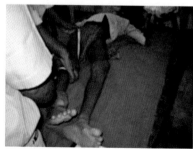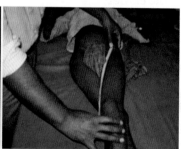

What is being shown in above figures?
Measurement of thigh segment on both the sides.

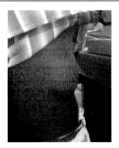

What is this condition?
Cold abscess.

How will you investigate this?
X-ray and MRI of spine.

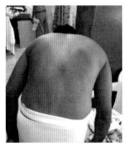 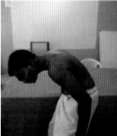 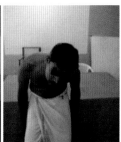

What is the diagnosis?
Ankylosing Spondylitis.

What biochemical test is typical of this condition?
HLA B-27.

What is the test to test mobility of spine?
Schober's test.

What is the earliest sign in the lumbar spine X-ray lateral view?
Filling of the anterior concavity of the vertebral body.

What are the orthopedic procedures you can do to help him?
Wedge correction osteotomy of the spine.
Total hip replacement.

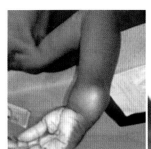 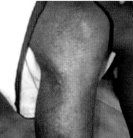 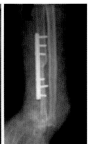 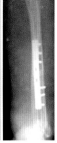

This 50-year-old man came with swelling in the distal forearm. First picture: He earlier had a surgery for the same site swelling 2 years back.

Picture 2: He has a scar in his right leg. His recent X-rays are shown in figure 3.

What is this condition?
Recurrent GCT distal radius.

What is that scar in the leg?
Donor area for the bone graft after the old distal radial resection.

What is the X-ray picture?
Plating done for fixing the graft to the residual radius shaft. Lesion affecting the grafted bone (fibula) also.

What could be the previous surgery?
Excision of GCT distal radius and reconstruction with a fibular grafting.

What is the treatment option now?
Amputation.

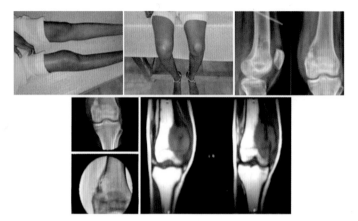

A 15-year-old girl had sudden onset of pain and swelling near her right knee joint

What is the possible diagnosis?
The X-ray of the girl with her MRI are shown.
Osteosarcoma of the distal femur.

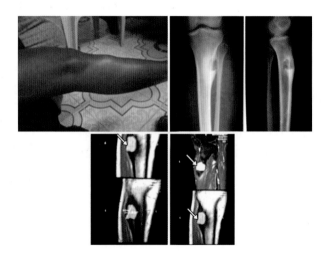

A 30-year-old lady came with swelling and pain of her left leg upper aspect.
Her X-rays and MRI are shown.

What is the lesion? What is your treatment option.

A GCT vartiant.

Curettage and bone grafting.

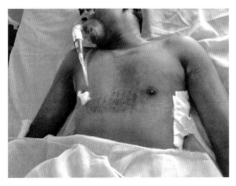

This 25-year-old boy was run over by a car.

What is the finding on the chest?

Tyre marks.

What radiological investigations you will order?

CT chest and abdomen to rule out the visceral injuries.

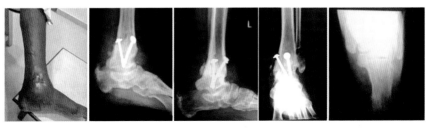

A 60-year-old gentleman a diabetic, had a surgery for a post-traumatic
arthritis of the ankle. He had discharging sinus from the medial wound.
His X-rays are shown. His current glycemic status is normal (HbA1c)

What was the possible surgery done?

Ankle arthrodesis.

What is this type of fixation is called?

Holz method.

What is the offending structure causing the problem?

The loosened washer and screw.

What is the common option of this above surgery?

Charnley's arthrodesis.

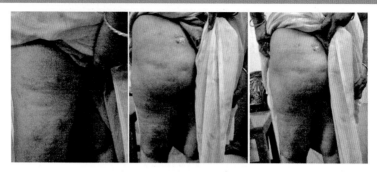

This 45-year-old lady was complaining of severe pain on the back of thigh and gluteal region for 2 days. The pain was unrelenting with NSAIDs like Aceclofenac 100 mg bids. Her lumbosacral X-rays were normal. Three days later, in inspection of the back and thigh this was the finding.

What do you find in gluteal region and the thigh?

She has developed herpetic vesicles

What is the significance of the direction?

It follows the direction of sciatic nerve.

How will you manage her?

She needs antiviral drugs, preferably referred to a skin specialist.

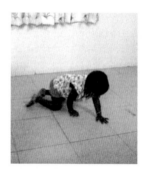

A 3-year-old child brought with complaints of not walking. The child also speaks only in monosyllables.

What questions will you ask in the birth history?

- Antenatal history
- Drugs /Anti-emetics/Anti-convulsant
- Diabetic mother
- Birth (normal/caesarian)
- Place of delivery at hospital or home/
- If delayed 2nd stage of labor was there
- If child cried immediately after birth.

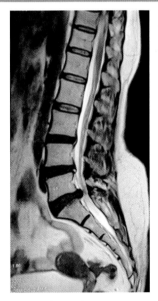

What is the radiological stage of the disease?
Disc extrusion.

Will conservation help in this case?
No, mostly the pain will persist even after conservation.

Which root will this disc compress?
S1 root.

Name two procedures for decompressing the root?
Minimally invasive discectomy, hemilaminectomy.

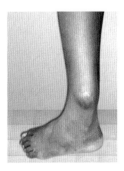

A 14-year-old boy came with a swelling of his leg near his ankle of 2 years duration. Occasional discomfort with no pain with mild shortening of his leg segment.

What is the possible diagnosis?
Exostosis.

Clinically from where this arises?
Postero - lateral aspect of leg possibly arise from fibula.

Why you tell this diagnosis?
Site-Bony swelling around the joint.
Age group – Skeletally immature age group.

What is the management?
X-rays to confirm the lesion.
If proved, extra periosteal excision.

Linked station

The following is the X-ray of the previous case?

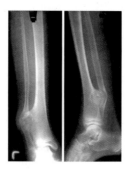

What is the lesion and from where this arises?
X-ray shows it actually arise from the tibia pressing on the fibula.
Abnormality of the host bone, e.g. Shortening, dysplasia.

Connected questions on ability to exam

What examination will you do?
Plane of the swelling arising from the bone.
Mobility of swelling
Movement of the near by joint.
Measurement of length of the bone for possible shortening.

Draw a skin incision for excision of this lesion in the upper fibula?

Exposure is for the nerve. Nerve is first protected. Then exostosis is resected.

Questions on Knowledge

Name the theories of origin of this swelling?
Theories of Exostosis – Periosteal defect theory and others.

Is this a tumor?
It is not a tumor. It is a developmental anomaly.

You have seen the photograph of the lesion and the X-ray. Why this swelling clinically appears larger than X-ray?
Cartilage cap is larger but does not throw a shadow in X-rays.

What are the complications of this swelling?
1. Mechanical block to movement of adjoining joint.
2. Adventitious bursa and pain.
3. Fracture of exostosis stalk and pain.
4. Malignant transformation.

What are the causes of pain in this condition?
1. Adventitious bursa.
2. Fracture of stalk.
3. Malignancy.

What is the malignancy that usually arises from this?
Chondrosarcoma (secondary).

Is it easy to identify the malignancy that arises from this lession?
It is difficult even for an experienced pathologist.

What are the radiologic-indicators of malignancy in this?
Haziness of outer cortex.
Irregular matrix inside the tumor.
Cartilage cap thickness. Measurement with MRI >6 mm

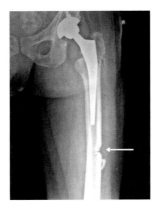

This 30-year-old man had a shaft of femur fracture and was treated with an inter locking nailing and implant exit. He was later found to have neck of femur fracture. He had this surgery. The arrow shows the original fracture site. **What you expect to happen on loading this limb?**
Fracture of the shaft of femur expected to happen below the prosthesis.

How would you avoid this complication?
Neck fractures should be seriously looked for in all cases of fracture femur, and addressed

How would you improve the present replacement?
By using a longer femoral stem component, or apply a locking plate

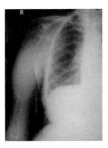

This is an X-ray of a 30-year-old male.

What is possibly the diagnosis of this condition?
Malignant bone tumour of right arm.

What is the investigation you will order?
MRI of the arm.

What will confirm the diagnosis?
By biopsy.

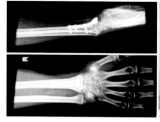 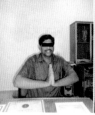 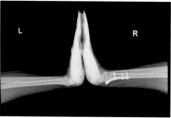

A 27-year-old male had fal from a two wheeler and a distal radial fracture. His postoperative pictures are shown.
What is the possible injury?
Volar Barton fracture.

What is the result?
Good function of the wrist as the X-rays are taken in maximum range of movement.

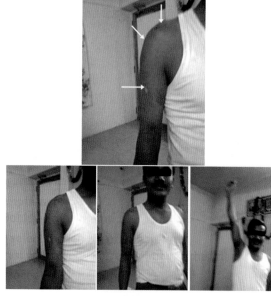

The above 3 arrows point areas corresponding to 3 scars which indicate 3 steps of the surgery of ILN of humerus
What are they?
1-Nail entry

2-Proximal locking
3-Distal locking.

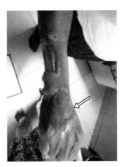

What is this flap?
Vascularized pedicle flap

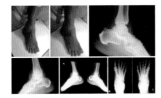

This patient has severe pain in the right ankle. He gives old history twisting injury to right ankle
What is your diagnosis?
Post-traumatic arthritis of the ankle.

What will be your treatment option?
Arthrodesis of the ankle.

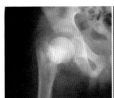 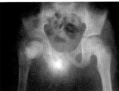 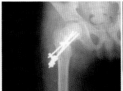

What is the diagnosis?
Fracture neck of femur in a child.

What is the procedure done?
Austin-Moore pin fixation.

What is the need for the immobilization done for this child in the last picture?
It will restrict the hip from moving till union.

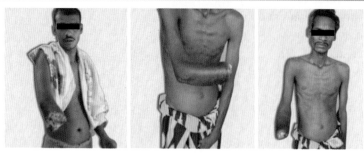

This is a common occupational injury in India.
What is it possibly due to?
Paddy thresher injury.

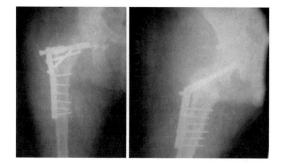

You are seeing two type of fixations for the same region of femur.
What is the advantage of first type of fixation over the second type and
What is the advantage of second type of fixation over the first type ?
More screws in proximal fragment in first. Hence, more control over shear of
upper fragment in first.
Chance of sliding compression (controlled collapse) in the second type
fixation (Figure 2).

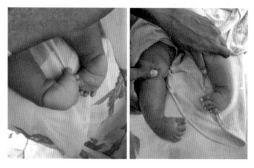

What is the condition?
Bilateral congenital talipes equinovarus.

What will be the affection of tibia?

Internal tibial torsion.

What is the main tendon-structure causing all the deformities and why?

Tibialis-posterior tendon, It is the tendon that is attached to all tarsal bones except talus.

Name the accepted theory of etiology of this condition? Other theories?

Abnormal uterine position theory of Hippocrates

Primary germ plasm talar defect

Primary soft tissue abnormality.

What are the differential diagnosis?

Myelomeningocele, Arthrogryposis, Tibial hemimelia. Poliomyelitis, Cerebral palsy, Constriction bands

What is the most common associated anomaly in system other than musculoskeletal system you will look for in this condition?

Urogenital.

Name only one fixation for each of these fractures.

No need to write the name of the fractures.

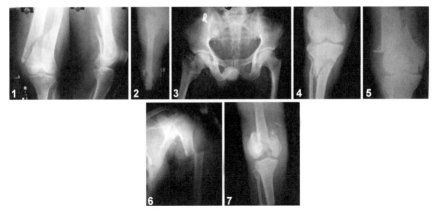

1. Long side plate with DCS/supracondylar nail, DFLCP
2. Interlocking nail
3. Dynamic hip screw system
4. Proximal tibial locking compression plate, hybrid fixation with Ilizarov
5. Dynamic condylar screw system
6. Interlocking nail humerus, board DCP
7. Intercondylar fracture fixed with cancellous screws and dynamic condylar screw system.

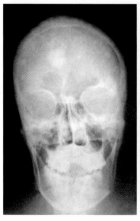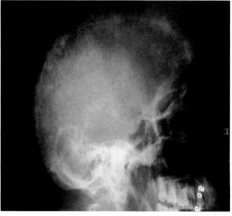

This in the skull X-ray of 56-year-old man lobe had severe pain in upper and lower limbs. He had a fracture of left thigh bone and was treated conservatively.

What is the disease?

Paget's disease.

Name systemic effect of this condition?

Congestive cardiac failure.

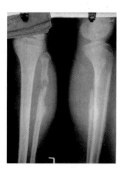

This 15-year-old child under retroviral therapy had a swelling over the outer aspect of left upper leg. These were his X-rays.

What is the diagnosis?

Osteomyelitis of fibula

What is the classification?

Cierny-MaderD diffuse type.
Immunocompromised host.

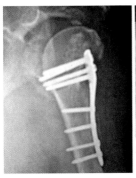 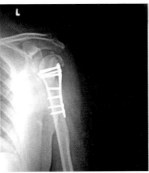 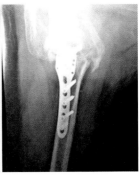

A 50-year-old man had a surgery for an injury to his left shoulder. These are his postoperative X-rays.

What is the implant?

Proximal humerus—Locking compression plate.

What has happened in the last picture and why?

A fragment is not purchased. Plate could have been placed higher.

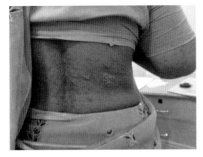

A case of severe loin pain which was unrelenting for 3 days and on clinical examination she has this finding? What is your clinical diagnosis?

Herpes zoster.

How will you manage this condition?

Should start antiviral drug—preferably by dermatologist.

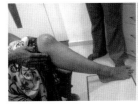 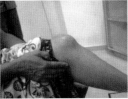

A 45-year-old lady had a fall at her house and developed gradual swelling in front of the knee.

What is the diagnosis?

Prepatellar bursitis.

What is the common name?
House maid's knee.

What is the definitive treatment?
Excision.

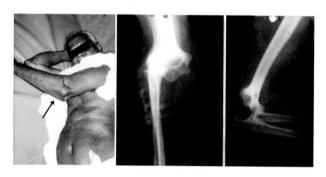

Instructions given to the Candidate

In the above pictures you are seeing a condition after a fall.
Name the condition?
Posterior dislocation of elbow.

How will you clinically confirm this?
Triceps standing out and taut.

How will you treat?
After confirmation with X-rays, closed reduction and plaster application is done in flexed position, under anesthesia.

What are the associated injuries?
Ulnar nerve injury.

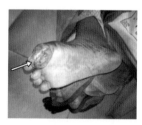

This 45-year-old lady came with this lesion (pointed with arrow) without pain. What is this condition?
Pressure ulcer.

What is the possible cause?
Diabetic peripheral neuropathy.

Name one imaging and one test to detect the predisposing cause, other than blood sugar?
X –ray of the foot.
Nerve conduction study.

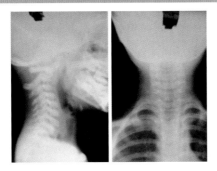

What do you observe in these X-rays?

Kyphosis of upper cervical spine.

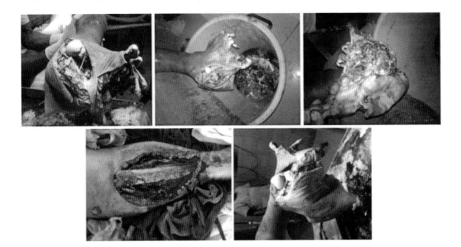

What has happened to this extremity?
Severe degree of crush injury.

How will you grade it for management purpose?
MESS (Mangled extremity severity score).

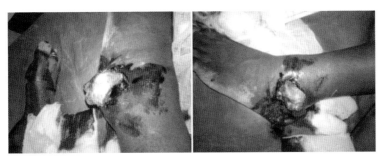

What has happened to the ankle?
There is open dislocation of the ankle

When will you reduce it and why?

The reduction should be done after debridement of the wound. If not the contamination will enter the ankle joint.

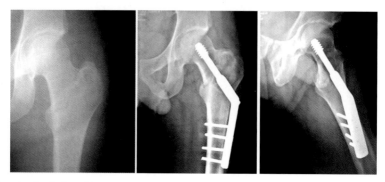

What is the injury?

Type 1 intertrochanteric fracture.

What is the fixation method?

Sliding hip screw.

What is the advantage of this system?

Controlled collapse and immediate partial weight bearing.

How you could have improved in this system?

Short barrel DHS side plate is better.

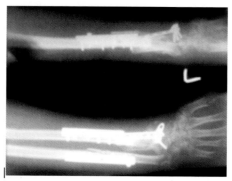

Name two possible reasons for such a fixation?

A second fracture.

Non-availability of implants.

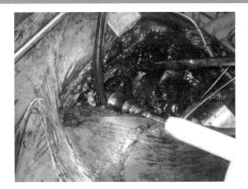

This is a hip surgery.
What is being done?
Acetabular reaming

In what direction the procedure should be done?
It is done with anteversion of 10 degree and 45 degree inclination to the body.

Before this procedure what will you ensure?
Real acetabulum is identified by removing the osteophytes.

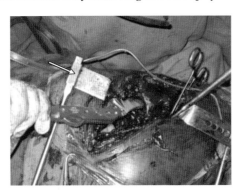

What is the procedure done?
Broaching or reaming for femoral component in a total hip arthroplasty or hemiarthroplasty.

What precaution before this procedure is taken and how it will be started?
Medullary canal is identified with an instrument like an IM nail reamer.

In what direction the procedure should be done?
Reaming started along the remnant of neck as lateral as possible and pointing towards medial femoral condyle.

What is the instrument pointed?
Charnley's self-retaining retractor for the hip.

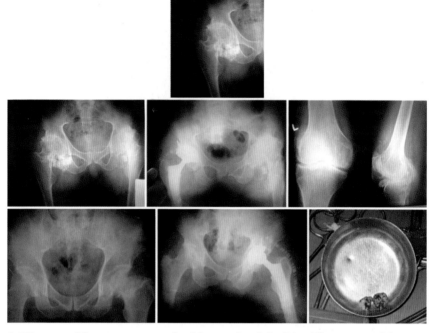

A 35-year-old man presented with a pain right hip. These were his preoperative and postoperative X-rays and during surgery the material seen in last figure was removed.

What is the diagnosis?
Synovial chondromatosis.

What is the pathological cause?
Synovial metaplasia.

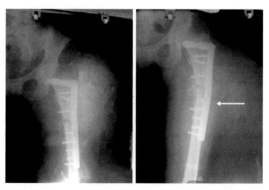

A 17-year-old, girl had an upper femoral fracture for which a DCS was done.
These are her early postoperative X-rays.
Between 1st and 2nd X-rays. What is the difference?
Bending of the plate.

What is the cause?
Premature weightbearing.

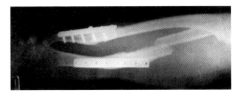

What has happened?
Second fracture after union of a fracture.

How it can be managed?
Plating without removing the previous fracture.

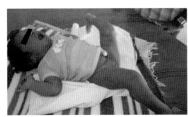 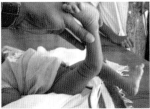

What is this condition?
Congenital dislocation of knee.

What is the status of anterior and posterior cruciate ligaments in these cases?
ACL/PCL are usually deficient.

What is the management if these cases present early?
Conservative applying plaster in flexed position.

What is the management if these cases present late?
Operative surgery- Quadriceps lengthening.

What would have been the mode of delivery of this child?
Caesarian section.

Why?
Because of breech presentation.

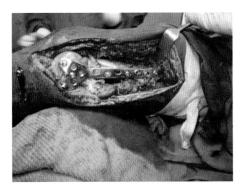

What is the implant used in the above procedure?
Condylar buttress plate.

What is the advantage of this over the DCS?
This removes less bone from the condyles of femur than the DCS.

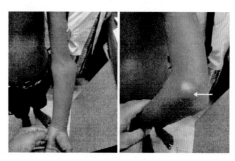

This **14-year-old boy came with this neglected trauma. The pointed structure moves with rotations of forearm.**

What is the possible structure pointed?
Radial head.

What is the possible diagnosis?
Monteggia fracture dislocation.

What is the other clinical test you do?
Measure length of the forearm segment.

How will you treat this boy?
X-ray confirmation.
Restoring ulna length.
Reduction of the radial head to its relation to the capitulum.

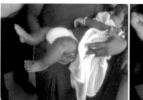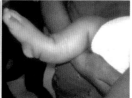

What is the diagnosis?
Posteromedial bowing of tibia (congenital).

What is the prognosis?
Good.

What is the reverse deformity is called?
Pseudoarthrosis of tibia.

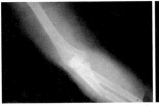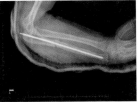

What is the fracture?
Upper ulnar shaft ftacture.

What is the implant used?
Talwalkar nail.

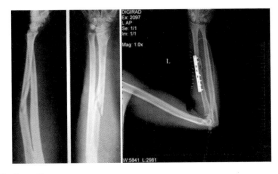

What is this injury?
Galleazi fracture dislocation.

What is the implant used?
Asian Narrow DCP

How will you tell this?
There is obliqueness in a screw with respect to the plate.

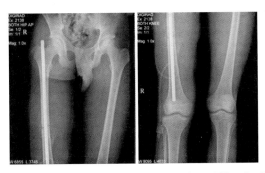

How will you measure the length of this implant if both the femora are fractured?
The distance between the tip of the little finger and the olecranon gives an approximate length of the nail.

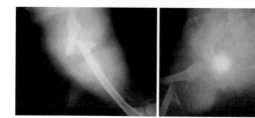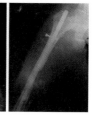

What is the deforming force of this proximal femur in first two figures?
Gluteus medius.

What is the implant used in last figure?
Interlocking nailing.

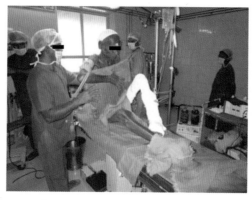

For the patient seen in the this picture, the left side lower limb is to be operated
How will you improve the position of this spinal to help your anesthetist?
You have completed one month special posting in anesthesia.
Bring the patient to the edge of the couch and hang the right lower limb down.
This will ease the spinal anesthesia.

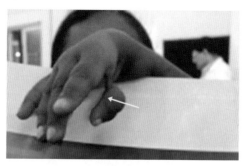

The thumb is hanging loose by a small skin
What is this condition?
There is intercalary loss of phalanx of thumb.

Is there any use of this finger?
Sometimes the skin of this finger can be used as a graft to cover injuries in the
neighboring fingers.

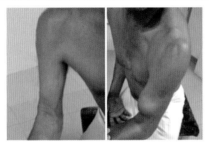

R   L

You are seeing the right and left arms of the same 60-year-old gentleman?
What is this condition?
Ruptured biceps tendon of left side.

What should have been the pre-existing symptom?
Shoulder pain.

How will you treat this condition?
In the old conservation.
In the young and active patients – resuturing and repair.

What is the appearance called?
'Popeye' biceps.

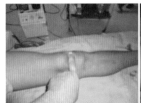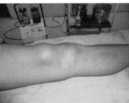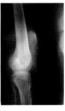

The patient had fallen 6 months back.
This is the palpatory finding.
What is this condition?
Nonunion of patella.

What are the palpatory findings you will ask the patient to do?
Straight Leg Raising.

What will you elicit when patient do SLR?
Extensor lag.

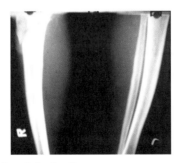

What is the lesion in the right leg?
Fracture seen in the upper leg.

Is this X-ray is enough?

No, the entire leg should be viewed (One joint above and one joint below).

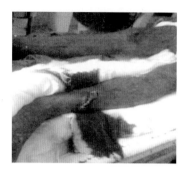

This 50-year-old diabetic had injury in a vehicular accident.
The left tibia was fractured and proximal end of the distal fragment was protruding out.

What is the treatment of choice?

Debridement.

External fixation – preferably Ilizarov ring fixator.

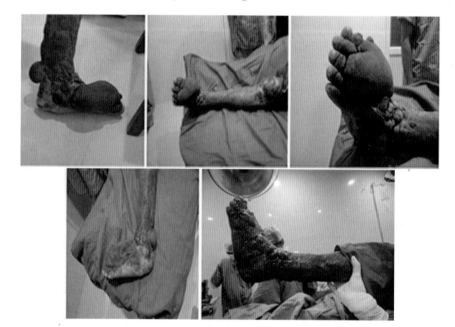

This 20-year-old male had an old crush injury while he was 5-year-old and skin grafting for that. Now he presents as shown in these figures?

What is this condition?

Unsightly lymphedema of the grafted area.

What is your advise?

Cosmetic debulking followed by pressure stockinette.

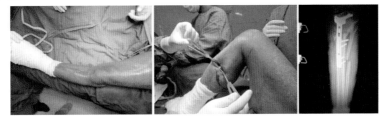

What is this condition—figure 1?
Varus of tibia

Why the incision is on the lateral side—figure 2?
The incision is to osteotomise the fibula.

What is the surgery done?
Corrective osteotomy of upper tibia to correct varus deformity.

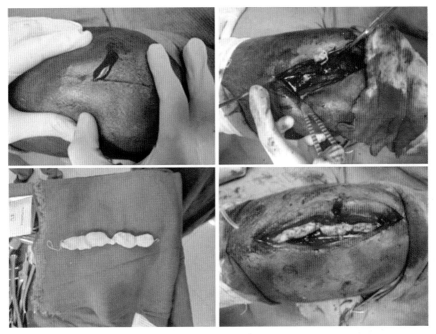

A 26-year-old had a internal fixation with infection shown in figure 1. The wound is being debrided in figure2. What is possibly being prepared in figure 3 and placed in the wound figure 4?
Antibiotic laden acrylic cement beads made on the table and kept in the wound.

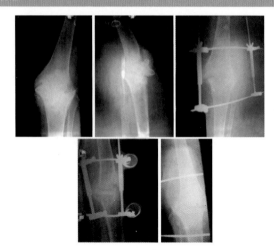

This 60-year-old had his total knee replacement done elsewhere which got infected and was referred here.

After debridement what is seen being kept in the joint space as seen in first two figures?

Antibiotic **L**aden **A**crylic **C**ement spacer (ALAC) kept in the joint space after debridement.

A particular apparatus applied in other figures. What is that?

Charnley's Compression Device.

What is the aim of this procedure?

Fusion of knee joint.

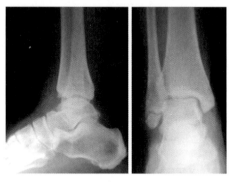

Where is the injury in fibula?

Infra syndesmotic fracture of lateral malleolus

What shall be the fixation method.

Tension band wiring

What is the prognosis?

If operated, the prognosis is good.

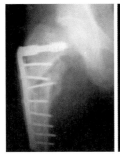
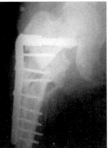

What is this injury?
Sub trochanteric fracture.

What is the implant used?
DCS.

What has happened in second X-ray?
Cut through of the DCS screw.

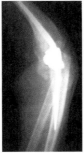
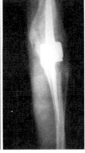

What is this surgery?
Total Elbow Replacement.

What are the types of joints available?
Cemented and Un-cemented.

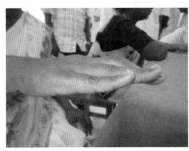
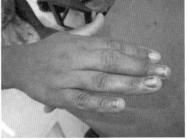

This 25-year-old had an injury while attempting to catch a cricket ball. What is the finding?
Middle finger PIP joint swelling.

What is the cause?
Post-traumatic arthritis—trauma.

If there is no history of this trauma then what are the common causes?
Gout → Metabolic
Rheumatoid arthritis → Autoimmune

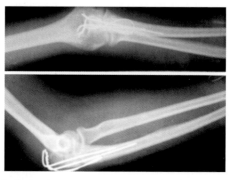

This 34-year-old lady had a surgery for elbow injury.
What is the lesion?
Olecranon fracture.

What is the surgery?
Tension band wiring.

There is no immobilization is it correct?
Yes. The basic principle in tension band wiring is early mobilization.

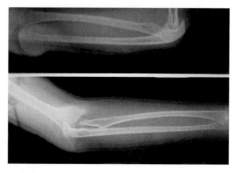

What is wrong with this?
A dysplastic elbow.

What will be the disability?
Instability.

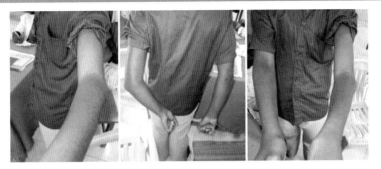

What is the deformity seen in the first picture?
Cubitus varus.

What is the movement being done in the second picture?
Internal rotation of the shoulder (left side).

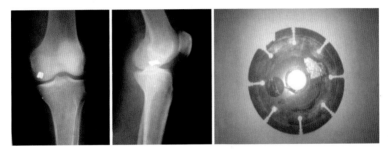

A 25-year-old presented with penetrating injury to the medial side of the right knee joint. The blade which was involved in the accident while cutting the marble slab is seen nearby.
How will you proceed?
Under image intensification control, the remnant piece of the blade (foreign body) can be removed.

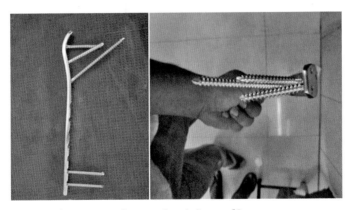

What is this implant? For what region it is used?
Locking compression plate for the proximal femur.

What is evident when the implant is seen from above?
It shows anteversion in the screw direction/non-parallel position of screws.

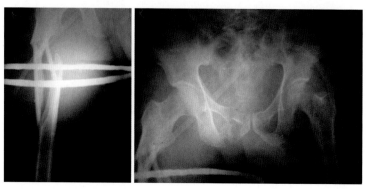

What classification you will use for this injury?
Russel-Taylor classification.

What are the implant effective in treating this fracture?
Interlocking nail/PFLCP, DCS system.

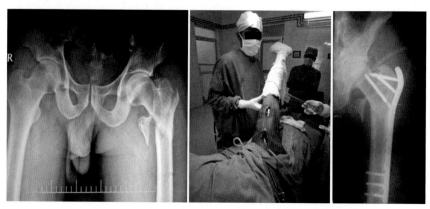

In this series of photos one procedure is described, what is that?
Sliding type of biological plating.

Its complications?
If plate is fixed without reduction then it will lead to non-union.

Why there are two incisions?
Sliding type of plating.

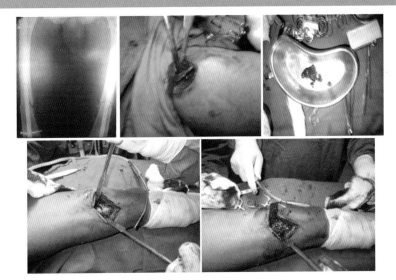

A postoperative X-ray is shown in picture 1, i.e. 4 months after a surgery.

What is the condition?

Bilateral fracture distal third shaft of femur, both fixed with an interlocking nail.

Second and third pictures show intraoperative photos of a surgery and the material taken during the surgery in the same patient from another site.

What is the possible surgery and what is the material taken?

Autologous bone graft harvesting and bone graft material.

What is possibly being done in the next picture?

The ununited fracture site of the right femur is exposed.

What is being done in the next picture?

The non-union site is packed with bone graft material.

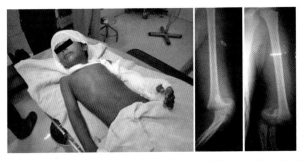

This 7-year-old had an elbow injury and immobilized. He also had severe pain in the forearm and elbow.

He also has severe pain, difficulty in moving the fingers especially extension.

What is the lesion?

Grade 3 supracondylar fracture.

What has he developed?
Compartment syndrome.

What one clinical sign you will elicit?
Stretch pain.

How will you objectively diagnose this condition?
Compartment pressure measurement.

What will be the treatment?
Fasciotomy followed by fixation.

What 2 main structures you need to release at wrist and elbow?
Flexor retinaculum.
Lacertus fibrosis.

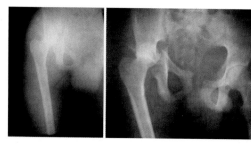

What is this injury?
Fracture acetabulum with dislocation.

What is the most common violence that causes this sort of injury?
Dash board injury.

What is the management in this case?
Closed reduction of hip dislocation and lower femoral pin traction.
Closed reduction of hip dislocation and internal fixation of the acetabulum.

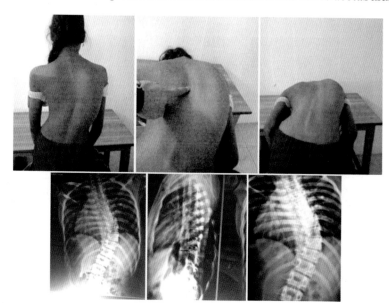

A 12-year-old girl has this deformity and she was able to stoop forward.

What is pointed in the 2nd picture and 3rd picture?
Structural scoliosis.
Rib hump.

How will you assess the flexibility of the spinal curve?
Right and left lateral bending AP view.
Lateral view—Hyperextension.

Name one another X-ray you will order ? and why?
X-ray pelvis—to find the skeletal age.

Name one another system you examine.
Respiratory system.

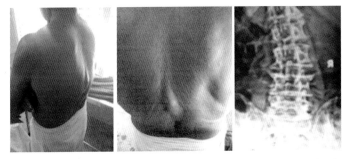

This 50-year-old who had Anti-Tubercular drugs for pain in the back and still has this finding.
Will ATT not correct this deformity?
ATT will control the disease, not necessarily correct this deformity.

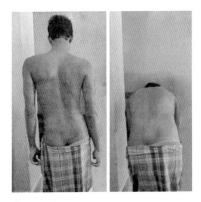

What is seen in first picture?
A list is seen in the spine.

What has happened to the finding seen in the first picture, in the second picture?
The list is reduced after stooping.

What is this called?
Sciatic scoliosis or non-sciatic scoliosis.

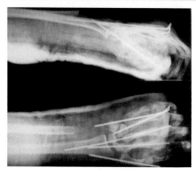

What is the possible fractures in this fixation?
Metacarpal fracture.
What are the other injuries seen?
Loss of distal ulna.

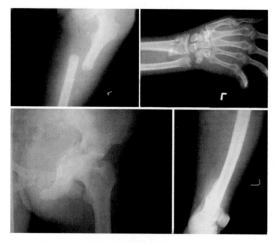

Name only one fixation for these fractures?
You no need to write any specific approaches.
A→Interlocking Nailing, B→External Fixator
C→Reconstruction plate, D→Interlocking Nailing /Supracondylar Nail.

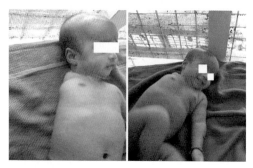

This child has a congenital problem.
What is your diagnosis?
Congenital agenesis of right upper limb.

What will be the disability when compared to an acquired condition of similar limb loss in adult?
Disability is lesser as the child gets used to the deficiency.

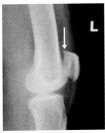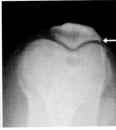

What are the marked findings?
Osteophyte of patella.

What will be the main disability of this individual?
Difficulty in climbing stairs.

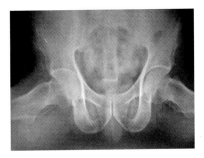

What is the view?
Frog lateral view of both hips.

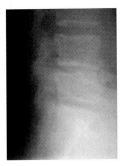

What is seen in this X-ray? What is your comment on sagittal relationship of the vertebrae?
Loss of lumbar lordosis.

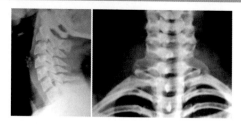

What is this condition?

Cervical rib left side.

How will you count the cervical vertebrae and the dorsal vertebra?

The transverse process of last cervical vertebra points downwards.

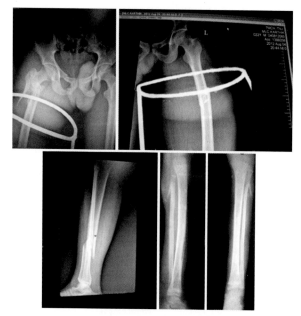

Diagnose A, B, C and D and mention treatment for each.

A → Russel-Taylor IB—reconstruction nail

B → Shaft of femur middle third-interlocking nail

C → Fracture both bones leg middle and distal third—interlocking nail of tibia

D → Upper third fibula fracture–conservation.

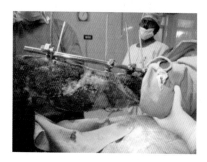

What are the problems in this limb of a 56-year-old diabetic male?

1. Raw area.
2. 2 pins in proximal and 3 in distal fragment.
3. Diabetes.

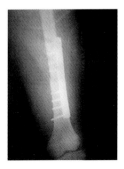

What is the fixation device?
A broad DCP.

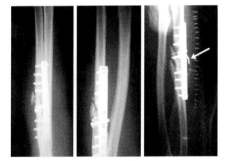

What is unusual in this fixation pointed?
A cerclage wire is applied.

What is its disadvantage?
It may cut through the bone.

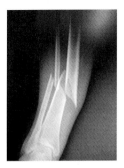

Are you satisfied? What is needed?
No, the entire leg need to be viewed.

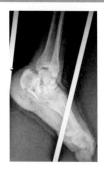

What is this injury?
Calcaneal fracture.

What are possibly these linear artifacts?
Rods of the Thomas splint.

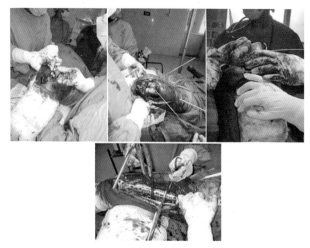

What is being done in an operation on the distal femur in figures 1, 2 and 3. What is exactly attempted.
Reconstruction of the distal femur fracture. Intra-articular element with K-wires.

What is the implant used?
Condylar buttress plate.

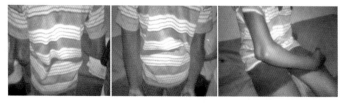

This is a boy with an old elbow problem seen from back, front lateral. What is the condition?
Neglected dislocation of elbow.

Which finding decided your diagnosis?
Taut triceps.

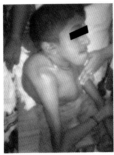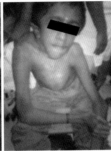

What is the facies you are seeing in this child?
Triangular facies.

What is this condition?
Osteogenesis imperfecta.

What is the classification?
Sillence classification.

What is the common cardiac problem?
Aortic incompetence.

What are the possible skeletal problems?
Pathological fractures and prompt healing with deformities.

What is the treatment done ?
Prophylactic nailing and fixations.

What prophylactic drug can be given?
No specific treatment.
Vitamin D and calcium can be given.
Oral MgO 15 g/kg will reduce the risk of fractures.

Can you see a typical facies in the illustrated picture?
Yes. It is the classic triangular face of type III Sillence.

Type	Genetic	Sclera	Severity	Fractures
I	AD	Deep blue	Mild	Easily heal
II	Sporadic/AR	Normal	Lethal	Multiple
III	Classic triangular face AR	Blue grey-lighter	Severe deforming Few survive to adulthood	Multiple fractures with joint laxity
IV	AD	Pale blue	Moderately severe	No fractures after adolescence

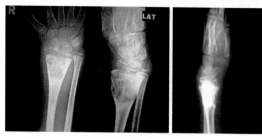

What is this condition? What is the treatment done?
ABC of the distal radius. Hydroxy-apatite filling after curettage of the cavity.

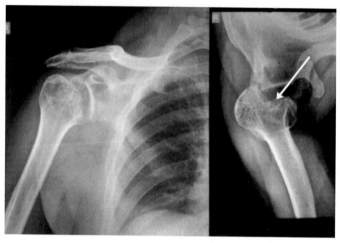

What is pointed?
Postero lateral defect in head of humerus

What shall be the primary cause of this lesion?
Recurrent dislocation of shoulder.

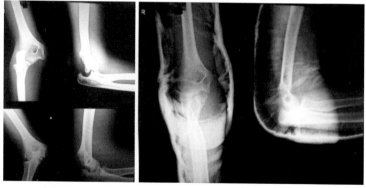

In the first picture you see a lesion.
In the next you see the picture of the same patient after treatment

What is the condition?
Dislocated elbow.

What is the treatment?
Closed reduction.

What will be one important function that will need to be checked after the reduction?
Ulnar nerve function.

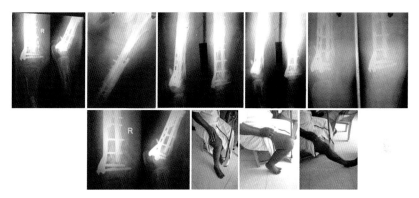

This 40-year-old fisherman in a vehicular accident 5 years back had a fracture of right thigh which was operated first. Then an additional implant and bone grafting was done to same fracture in another centre. Patient had union and was walking for past four years with these implants 1 month back he had one more injury. This needed a third surgery and a third implant to be applied on the femur.

What are the possible surgeries and implants?
1. Inter-locking nail.
2. Broad DCP with bone grafting.
3. Condylar buttress plating.

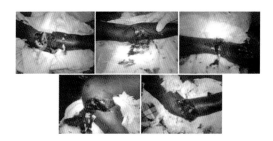

Above are appearances of a multiple injured patient

How will you grade these injuries?
MESS.

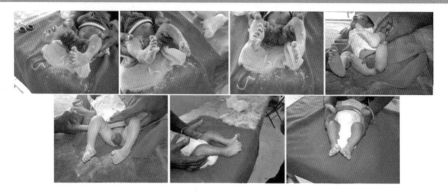

This is the last plaster of a CTEV child

What is the result?
Good.

What scoring will you use?
Pirani.

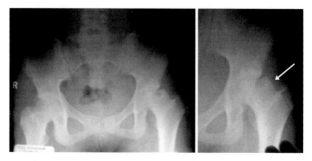

What is pointed in the figure?
Hinged abduction.

What will not be useful?
Varus derotation osteotomy.

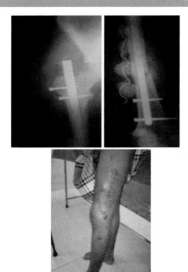

A case of infected interlocking nailing.

What is seen in the above pictures?

1 and 2 pictures the fracture was debrided and Antibiotic Laden Acrylic Cement is kept.

You are seeing the present scar position. What it indicates?

The patient's present scar position suggests that the infection is under control.

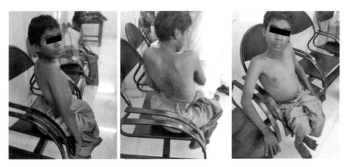

This 12-year-old had difficulty in walking since childhood. He has deformity since early childhood.

What are the questions you will ask in history regarding course of this disease.

Consanguinous marriage.

H/o poliomyelitis /fever/fall/ immunization/

Progression or improvement of the weakness.

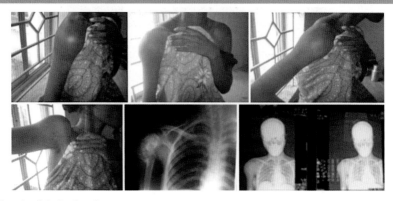

What is this lesion?
Chondrosarcoma of the proximal humerus.

How it affects the range of movement of the shoulder?
It mechanically blocks abduction and flexion.

What is the treatment?
MRI-Core needle biopsy, wide excision and reconstruction.

What chemotherapy will you give?
Chemotherapy is not useful.

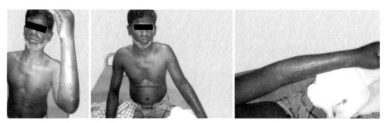

This patient was operated for a fracture both bones of forearm.
He was asked to do this in the ward. He will be sent to home with a plaster.

What is this method of immobilization?
Perkin's delayed splintage.

What is the advantages?
More gain in the range of movement as initial stiffness is prevented.
The mobilization is supervised so that the chances of increased loading do not occur.

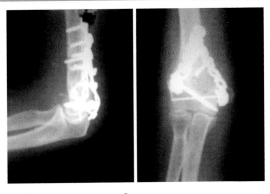

What are the implants you can see?

Reconstruction plates.

Malleolar screw, K-wire

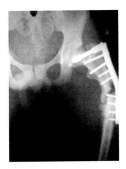

What is the best way to treat this 17-year-old boy who put weight before advice if you donot have a image intensifier in your theater.

1. Maintain the DCS screw.
2. Reapply another barrel plate, with longer side plate (12H or 14H)
3. Bone grafting.

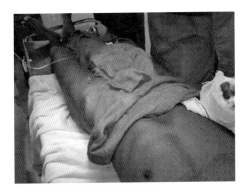

What is done?

A needle is passed perpendicular to the skin, possibly lateral to the femoral artery.

What are the possible procedures?
Femoral nerve block.

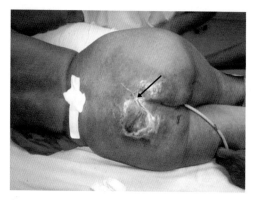

Why the patient is put in this position? What is the pointed lesion? Why dressing is done elsewhere?
This patient is positioned in lateral position for surgery.
The pointed lesion is a bed sore.
It is the plaster for the spinal injection site.

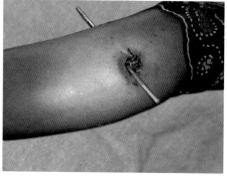

What is this?
Pin tract infection.

What is the name of this pin?
Steinman pin.

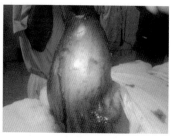

What is being done? In what position?
The left thigh is prepared in supine position.

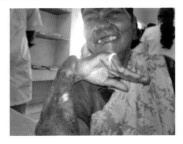

What is the diagnosis?
Old crush injury forearm.

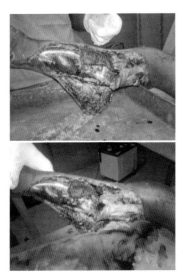

This is a crush injury to the calf region. There was no bony injury

What are the steps of your management?
Debridement.
Blood transfusions,
Antibiotics, loose stitches and
primary skin grafting.

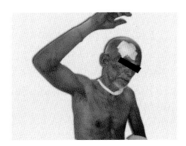

This maneuver rules out certain injuries.

What are they?
This rules out major proximal upper limb injuries.

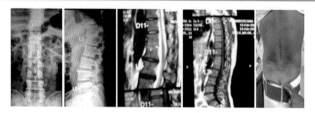

Note the scar and the MRI.

What is your diagnosis?
Old healed TB spine with drained cold abscess.

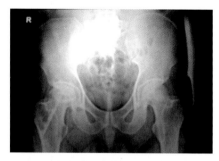

This 25-year-old occasional alcoholic came with pain hip right side. After 2 types of investigations, he was operated. This is his postoperative X-ray.

What is the surgery?
Core decompression and fibular grafting.

What are those investigations?
MRI/Tc-99m scan.

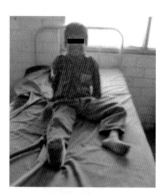

You are seeing this boy in the ward. He was applied a below knee slab on the right side. What is your inference?
The boy is walking with the slab.

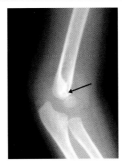

What is the pointed region is called?
Tear drop.
It corresponds to the supracondylar region.

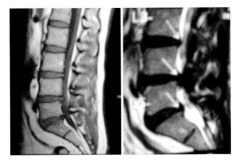

What is the lesion?
L4/5 disc.

What root will it compress?
L5 root.

What muscle is expected to be weak?
Extensor hallucis longus.

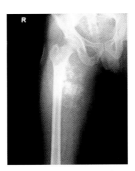

25-year-old male who was having no symptoms previously had a swelling for past three months and pain for the past 15 days.
What is the radiological finding?
Pop corn like calcification of the mass.

What is the diagnosis?

Chondrosarcoma.

What is the type, and why?

Primary.

There is no evidence of a pre-existing lesion like an exostosis.

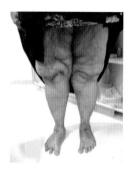

55-year-old underwent a surgery for pain knee both sides.
What is the possible surgery?

Total knee replacement.

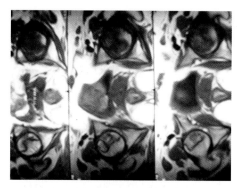

45-year-old alcoholic had pain both hips. He has this MRI findings? What is the most common diagnosis?

Avascular necrosis of hip.

Name one important test you will order?

Technetium-99m scan.

Name one procedure you will do?

Core decompression.

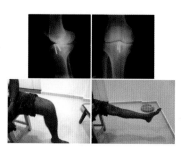

What is the possible surgery?
Anterior tibial spine avulsion.

What is attached to the fractured fragment?
ACL

What is the result of this surgery?
Good.

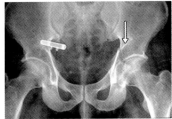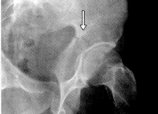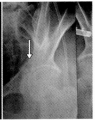

What view is in the first film?
Pelvis AP.

What is the second view?
Iliac view.

What is the third view?
Obturator view.

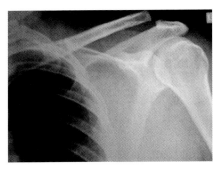

What is the mode of injury to this patient?
Fall on to the point of the shoulder.

Why clavicle is separated/from acromion?
It was stopped by the rib cage, while still acromion is moving.

What is the grade in this lesion?
Grade 2.

What is the classification?
Rockwood classification.

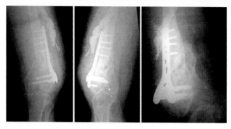

Name 3 possible problems in this patient?
Infection- antibiotic beads are seen.
Un-united fracture.
Persisting deformity.

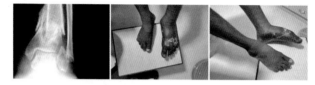

This 50-year-old male had an injury of left leg 4-month back with indigenous treatment.
What is the finding?
Swelling of left foot, shiny skin, trophic changes of nails
Left side foot.

What is the condition of fracture in X-ray?
Malunion of the tibia and displace lateral malleolus.

Clinically what is the disease?
Reflex sympathetic dystrophy.

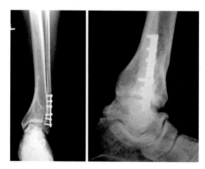

This 30-year-old man had injury to his left leg and surgery for that injury 6 years back.
He now has pain in the ankle.
What is the diagnosis?
Malunited fracture distal tibia.

Will implant removal reduce his pain?
No.

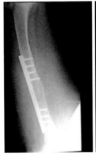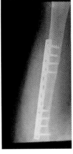

What is this plating is called?
Wave or bridge plating. (Biological plating)

How it is different from the regular plating?
Not disturbing the fracture. No screws near the fracture site.

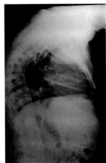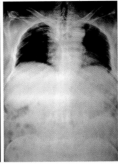

What is striking in the lateral view?
Osteoporosis and kyphosis.

What one diagnostic test you will do in urine?
24 hours urinary calcium excretion.

What is the treatment options?
Calcitonin nasal spray.

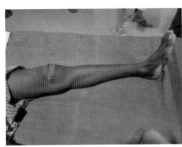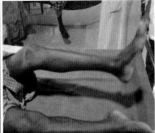

In these two snaps patient is asked to raise a straight leg
Where is the lesion?
Rupture of the quadriceps tendon. (Extensor lag)

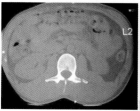 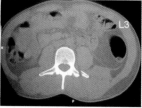 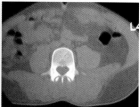

In the three images shown above, what are the lesions?
Fracture transverse processes of L2, 3 and 4 of left side.

What is the cause for concern in this case?
Shock due to increased bleeding.

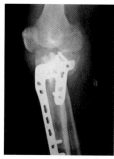 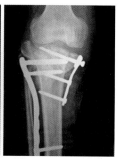

What are the implants? What is this surgery?
Locking compression plates on the lateral side and posteromedial side of upper tibia.

What has happened to the medial side plate?
Loosened, one screw is in the joint.

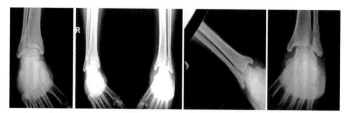

What is the special view the last picture show? How it is done?
Mortise view. It is done by taking an AP view in 20 degrees internal rotation.

What is the fracture?
Oblique fracture of the lower fibula.

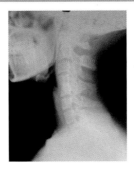

What is unique in this X-ray?
Block vertebra.

What is the problem of the other vertebra due to this?
Degeneration.

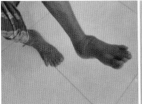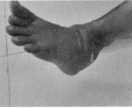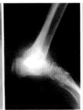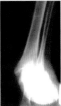

A 50-year-old male had an injury to the left ankle 6 months back. There was tenderness in the joint line. His X-rays are available.
What is the diagnosis?
Post-traumatic arthritis.

What are the investigations required now?
CT Scan and MRI of the ankle.

What is the possible surgical option?
Fusion of the ankle.

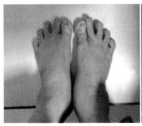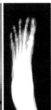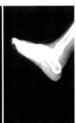

What is unusual about the second toe?
The second toe is deviated to the great toe.

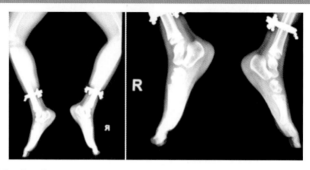

What is this view?
Lateral view of the leg ankle and the feet in plantar flexion.

What is that needs to be ruled out?
Congenital vertical talus.

Name one thing that could have been done before taking these films?
The anklet could have been removed.

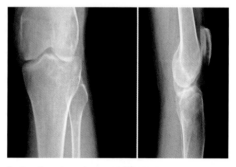

A 30-year-old male had pain after a fall and was not able to walk. What is the lesion?
Minimally displaced fracture of lateral condyle of femur.

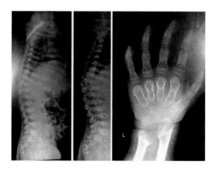

What is this condition?
Mucopoly saccharidosis.

Name 2 of them?
Hurler's disease, Morquio's disease.

What are the abdominal organs involved?
Hepatosplenomegaly.

What are the tests you will order in urine-biochemistry?

Chondroitin sulfate	Hurler's disease
Heparan sulfate	Keratin sulfate – Morquio's disease.

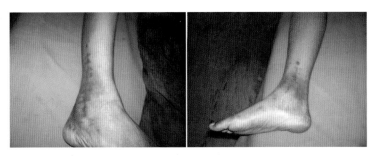

What is the most probable surgery done on this patient?
Bimalleolar fracture fixation.

If you have only one X-ray film, which view will you do for this patient?
Mortise view of the ankle.

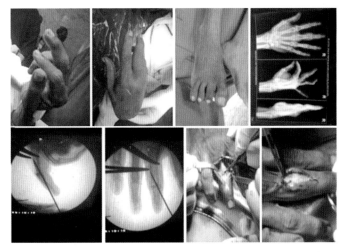

This 60-year-old occasional alcoholic, a non-smoker had pain and stiffness of his right middle finger.

What is the possible cause in this condition?
Gout.

Name one blood investigation you will order?
Uric acid.

What is the possible surgery being done on him?
Fusion of the involved PIP joint.

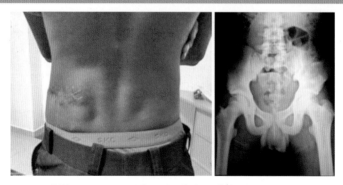

This 16-years-old boy came with pain left side hip. He had surgery on his left buttock.

What is the possible diagnosis?

Osteomyelitis of left iliac bone.

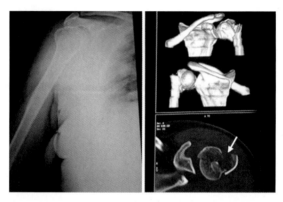

These are the X-rays and the reconstruction CT of a 40-year-old man who presented 14 days after injury. What are his 2 main problems?

Comminution.

Late presentation.

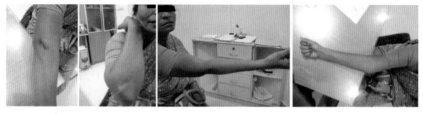

You are seeing a scar on the lateral aspect of right elbow on this lady. She did not have any injury. She has a good range of movement. She had surgery for the pain in the elbow 5 years back.

What are the possible causes of this surgery?

Tennis elbow.

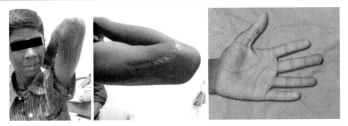

You are seeing 2 scars, postoperative status in this child.
What are the possible surgeries done on this child?

1. Supracondylar fracture humerus.
2. Ulnar nerve transposition- anteriorly.

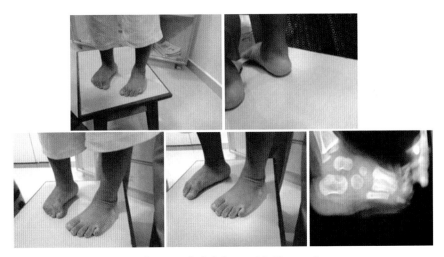

You are seeing a case of treated clubfoot with Ponseti.
What is the result?

Forefoot adduction – still not corrected.

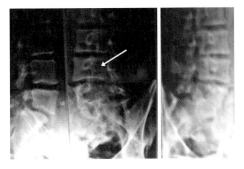

What does the arrow points?

The isthmic region.

What part of the terrier dog the pointed part forms?

The neck.

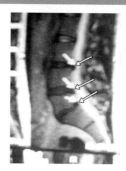

What is this investigation?
MRI of LS spine.

What are the levels the small arrows point in this picture?
L3/4,L4/5,L5/S1 Discs.

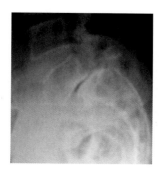

What is this condition?
L5/S1 listhesis.

How will you manage this condition if there is severe pain in one of the lower limb?
Traction for 6 weeks.
If no response, S1 root decompression and fusion.

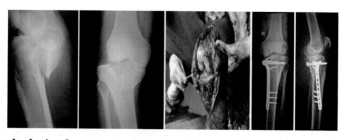

What is the lesion?
Medial condyle fracture of tibia.

What is the fixation?
Locking plate fixation.

What is the most important step of this surgery?
Holding the posteromedial fragment with a scew.

Mention one preoperative investigations that might be useful.
Reconstruction CT of knee joint.

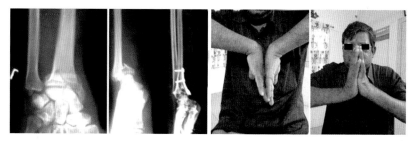

What are the movements seen in last 2 figures?
Volar flexion and dorsiflexion.

What is this lesion?
Volar Barton's fracture.

What is done?
Buttress plating.

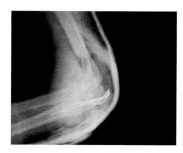

What is seen in this view?
Tension band wiring

What is paradoxical here and why?
The plaster of Paris.
The TBW is meant to mobilize the elbow but plaster of Paris is applied.

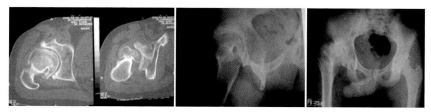

What is this investigation?
X-ray and CT of the hip.

What is the diagnosis?
Coxa magna , most probably Perthes.

How will you treat this condition?
THR.

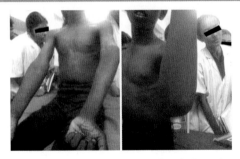

What is the deformity of elbow? Where is the deformity- in the humerus or forearm? Why?

Cubitus varus.

On flexion deformity dissapperars so deformity is in humerus.

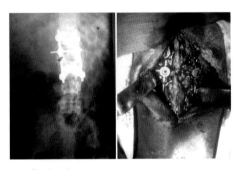

What is this fixation device?

Moss Miami system.

How many columns of spine it fixes?

Three columns → anterior, middle and posterior.

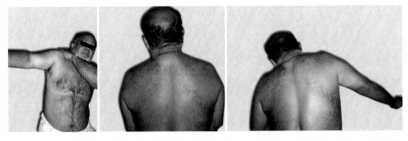

This 50-year-old man had a fall in vehicular accident. He could not abduct his shoulder.

What is the possible injury?

Rotator cuff injury.

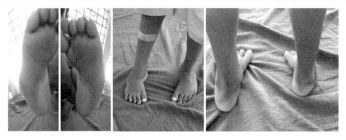

This is a postoperative condition of a CTEV.

What is the result?

The forefoot adduction is still not corrected.

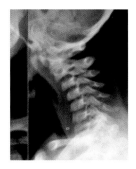

What is the normal alignment of the cervical spine?

Lordosis.

Is this X-ray normal?

No, this cervical spine is in kyphosis.

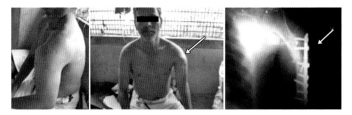

This 40-year-old man had a surgery for an injury of his left arm. His X-ray also is given.

What is his problem now?

Loosening of the implant

What are possible causes for this?

Less screws proximally.

Premature loading of the limb.

Osteoporotic bone.

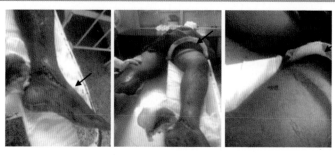

What is the name of the pointed appliance used to rest the lower limb?
Thomas splint.

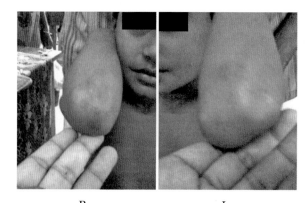

R   L

You are seeing the right and left elbows of the same child. What is being compared?
The three bony points of the elbow are compared.

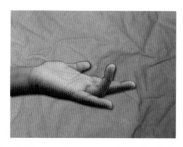

This 45-year-old diabetic has pain on flexing the left middle finger beyond this level.
After full flexion he can only extend the finger with a snap. What is this condition?
Trigger finger.

What is the pathology?
Tenovaginitis of the FDP.

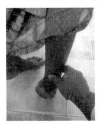

This 40-year-old is asked to stand on the toes. What is the structure palpated?
Tendo-Achilles.

What was the patient is asked to do?
Stand on the toes.

What is the possible diagnosis, expected to be ruled out?
Tendo-Achilles rupture.

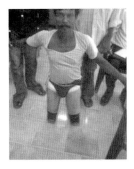

This 40-year-old had lost his both lower limbs in a rail accident.
What is the name of this prosthesis?
Stubbies.

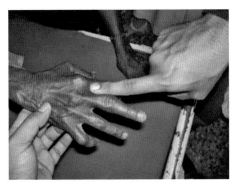

This is a lady with symmetric small joint pain. What is being demonstrated?
Ulnar deviation of the fingers.

What are the causes for this?
Shape of the phalangeal head, ulnar side positioning of the extensor tendons, reducing length of the metacarpal towards 5th metacarpal.

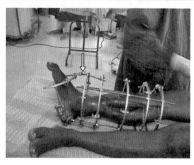

Name the device applied on the lower limb?
What is the pointed structure?
The foot assembly to correct the equines deformity, by III Ilizarov method.

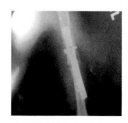

What is wrong with this fixation?
Plate is offset.
A longer plate should have been applied.

Mark the skin incision for a specific surgery.
Hemiarthroplasty by posterior approach.
Hip biopsy
Anterior decompression of spine.
Anterolateral decompression of spine
Bone graft harvesting
Total hip replacement
Total knee replacement
Fibular plating
Tension band wiring of medial malleolus
Radial head excision
Wrist fusion
Shoulder proximal humerus fracture fixation
Humerus shaft fracture anterior exposure
Radial nerve exploration
Elbow fixation
Forearm fracture
Femoral shaft fractures
Tibial shaft fracture
Posterolateral bone grafting
Fasciotomy for the forearm fracture
Fasciotomy for the leg injury.

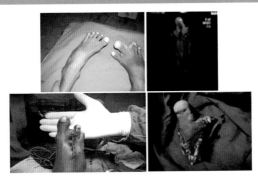

This 12 year old boy presented with the clinical picture as shown in 1st picture. He had assessment included a search for any other evidence of neuro-fibromata, MRI of the part and an arterial Doppler. He also underwent surgery which is shown in 3rd picture. The 4th picture shows the resected specimen.

What is the clinical diagnosis?

Localised gigantism.

What will be the cause?

Plexiform neurofibroma of foot involving the second and third toes.

What will be his problem, he will be having while going to school?

Inability to wear shoes.

Both cosmetic and functional problem.

What is the surgery done?

Ray amputation of the toes.

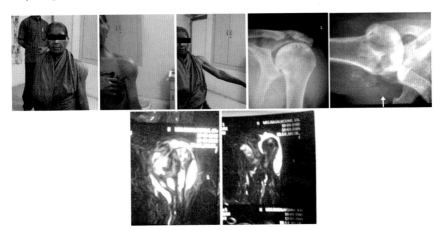

This 60-year-old lady had pain and swelling in the left shoulder. There was crepitus on palpating the swelling. She could actively move the shoulder but all movements especially the abduction was restricted.Her blood investigatons blood sugar and ESR were normal. Her X-rays and MRI are seen.

What is the possible diagnosis?
Synovial chondromatosis.

What is the pointed structure?
Cartilaginous loose bodies.

How will you confirm the diagnosis?
Synovial biopsy.

What will be seen in biopsy? or What is the pathology?
Cartilaginous metaplasia in the synovium.

What is the treatment?
Synovectomy.

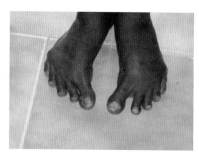

What is this condition?
Hallux varus.

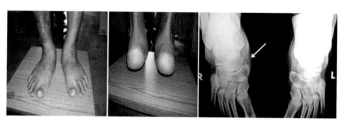

This 40-year-old male had pain over the medial part of the foot especially the navicula area-more on standing for more than half an hour.
What is this condition?
Bilateral flat feet.

What is the patient asked to do in the second figure and why?
Lift his heel to see if the long plantar arch is formed.

What tendon rupture can cause similar picture?
Tibialis posterior tendon rupture.

What is the finding in the X-ray?
Bilateral flat feet with accessory navicula which can even be unilateral. Flat arch laterally.

What is the candidate expected to look for?
Candidate should.

1. Look for flattening of the medial arch.
2. Ask the patient to stand on toes.

What is the treatment modalities?

Wax bath

Intrinsic muscle strengthening exercises to feet

Medial arch support.

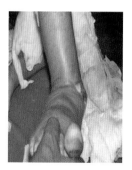

A case of open ankle dislocation in a diabetic patient.
What are the requirements of this patient?

Needs debridement, glycemic control, and antibiotics, skeletal stabilization

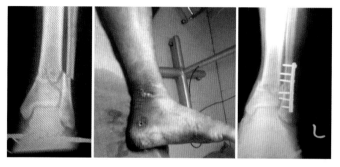

This is an injury in a 45-year-old with open wound—
initially managed with calcaneal pin traction.

What are the fractures?

Pilon fracture and distal fibular fracture.

What will be the line of management?

Due to poor skin condition, treated with fibular plating.

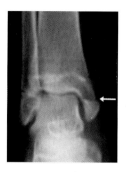

What is seen in this X-ray?

Avulsion injury of medial malleolus.

Is this X- ray is enough?

For the lateral side the entire fibula should be X-rayed to rule out a fracture.

What structure will cause non-union of the pointed lesion?

Invagination of periosteum into the fracture.

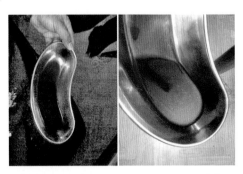

This is the aspirated blood from hemarthrosis of knee. A closer view shows some small shiny things is floating on the surface.

What are these "small shiny things"?

Fat globules.

What is their origin?

Marrow fat.

What is the inference?

Intra-articular fracture.

What should the surgeon do?

Look carefully at the X-rays again. If needed must do an MRI.

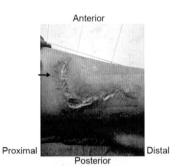

In this incision of letting out an hematoma of the thigh, what is your comment on the incision, especially the site marked by arrow?

The marked area is a transverse incision in the thigh, which could have been avoided.

The limb incisions preferably be longitudinal.

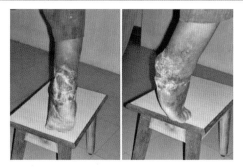

What is this painless lesion that has arised from an old scar?
Marjolin's ulcer.

How will you proceed?
Painless ulcer on a healed scar. Biopsy is warranted.

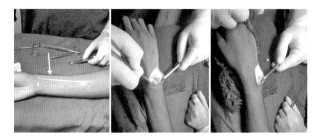

What is the structure being dissected?
Palmaris longus is brought out from a proximal incision.

What is the possible indication?
Stabilization of the distal instability of ulna.

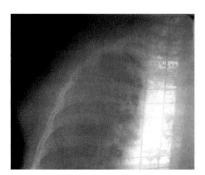

What do you see in this X-ray?
There is no scapula or shoulder joint.

What is the inference?
Either congenital absence of right upper limb or hind quarter amputation.

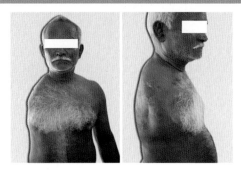

This is the patient whose X-ray was posted in your previous station.
Now what is your diagnosis?
Forequarter amputation done for possible malignancy of right upper limb.

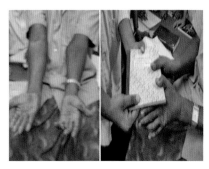

What is being tested?
Book test- adductor pollicis.

What is the observation?
Flexion of the IP joint of the thumb.

What is the inference?
Adductor pollicis is weak.
It is substituted by flexion of the IP joint of the thumb by FPL which is supplied by median nerve.

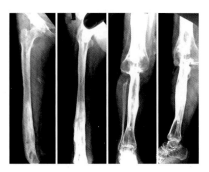

These X-rays are of a patient who had bone transport done for a tumor.
Where should have been the tumor?
Upper tibia.

What should have been the site of corticotomy?
Lower femur.

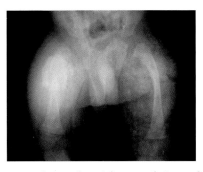

A 2-month-old infant was brought with complaints of not moving the left lower limb. Child was not taking feeds.
This was the X-ray.
What is your diagnosis?
Osteomyelitis of femur in a child.

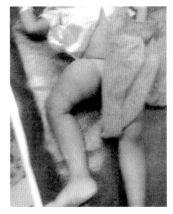

This 2½-year-old girl fell from a two wheeler and was brought with severe swelling of left thigh with inability to move her right lower limb. She had turmeric applied over the thigh.
What is the possible diagnosis?
Right side femur fracture.

What should be the immediate line of treatment?
Traction and Blood transfusion.

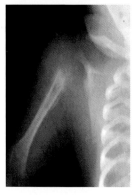

A one year-old-child was brought with complaints of not moving the right upper limb with severe swelling of right shoulder.
What is your differential diagnosis?
Septic arthritis of infancy
Osteomyelitis of upper humerus.

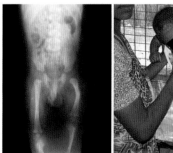 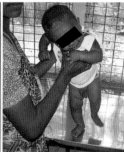 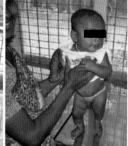

What is the diagnosis?
Congenital shortening of femur (proximal focal femoral deficiency) of left side

What is the classification?
Atkin's classification.

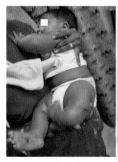 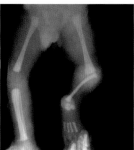 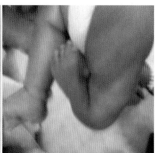

This child has short deformed left lower limb.
What is the skeletal problem?
Absent tibia—Tibial hemimelia.

How will you investigate and manage?
Confirm with X-rays and ultrasound a if there is a tibial analogue.
Amputation and rehabilitation.

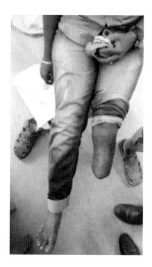

What is this?
A below-knee amputation stump

Where the fibula is cut in relation to tibia?
1 inch above the tibia

What is the immediate method to make this person walk after surgery?
Immediate postoperative prosthesis.

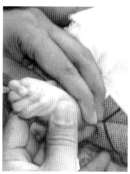 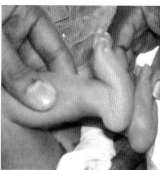 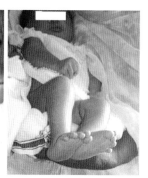

A child with Multiple congenital deformities is shown with the hand and feet findings.
What is the finding in hand?
Multiple congenital deformities thumb in palm.

What is the finding in the feet?
Rocker bottom feet.

What is the possible diagnosis?
Edward-patau syndrome.

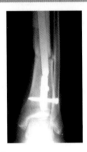

This is an X-ray of a patient who was operated 4 months back. What is your diagnosis?

Broken nail.

Name two possible causes?

- Leaving a hole free-a stress riser
- Premature weightbearing.

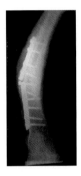

Broken plate-

Where was the break?

At the site of a scew hole.

What is the probable reason?

Probably due to premature weight bearing.

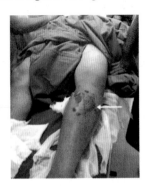

What are these lesions in a fracture both condyles of tibia?

Blisters after a fracture both condyles of tibia.

What important radiological investigation will you order other than the X-rays?

Venous Doppler.

What is the method of fixation you will do?

Minimally invasive plate osteosynthesis or hybrid fixation

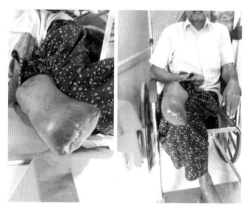

This is a 50 year old diabetic whose leg was amputated due to uncontrolled infection of leg .

In the next picture, you are seeing the close up of the stump.

Name two points that are not desirable about the stump end?

Scar is unhealthy.

There is dog ear in the ends – instead of conical end for fitting a prosthesis.

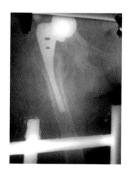

This is an old neck of femur fracture operated by routine posterior approach.

What are the problems and causes?

This is a case of loosened and dislocated prosthesis.

Causes → Uncemented implant AMP as holes are seen.

What additional procedure should have prevented this?

Adductor release should have been done for this old neck fracture.

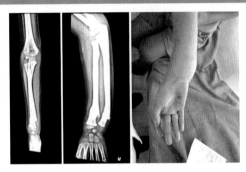

A 3-year-old boy had a fall and native treatment for the same.
What is the diagnosis?
Malunion distal fore arm
- Questions to the candidate
- To assess the ability to exam.

Can you clinically tell whether this fracture has united or not?
Expected outcome.
Candidate - Greets explains gets consent and undress adequate enough.
- Palpates for the radial head. Rotates the forearm holding the distal forearm
- If he feels the head rotating then confirms-Tests for transmitted mobility if present tells-union.
  If not–tells not united.

What will be the treatment?
Corrective osteotomy, realignment and fixation.

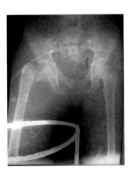

What is wrong with this?
Wrongly applied Thomas splint.
Its ring did not touch the ischial tuberosityt—see also the associated fracture of right pubis.

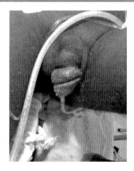

What is the lesion?
Paraphimosis.

What is the possible reason for this?
Failure to pull the prepuce forward after catheterization.

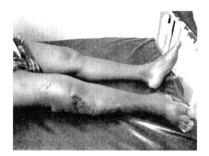

This 20-year-old had a fasciocutaneous flap done for a knee injury 5 years back.
Now has severe swelling of the entire leg.
What is the diagnosis?
Lymphedema of old flap area.

What is the diagnosis you should rule out?
Should rule out a deep vein thrombosis.

How will you start treatment?
Treatment is strict elevation.
Broad-spectrum antibiotics.
Anti-edema measures.

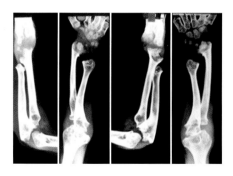

X-ray of forearm and elbow of a patient.

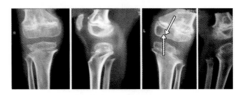

Preoperative X-rays of knee of the same patient.

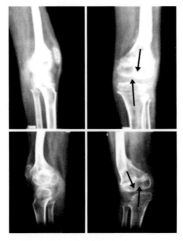

Postoperative X-rays of knees of the patient.

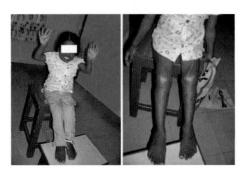

Girl after deformity correction

What should be the condition?
Morquios disease.

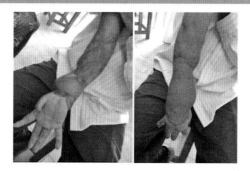

What is this?
Abdominal flap.

What should be the reason for this condition?
Crush injury of right forearm.

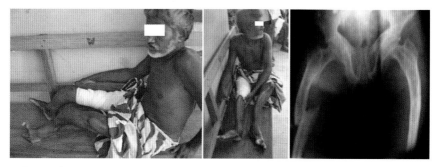

What is this condition?
Osteomalacia

What is the typical radiological appearance in pelvis marked?
Champagne glass-pelvis.

This 45-year-old male had has pain in the knee (anterior and posterior aspect of his right knee.

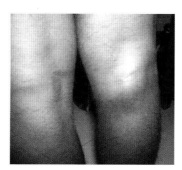

He had difficulty in squatting. This cystic swelling lesion in popliteal region, becoming less prominent on flexion and, more prominent on extension.

Associated with degenerative joint disease of knee.

What is the swelling?

Popliteal cyst.

How will you treat if patient is less than 6 years

Observe.

What is the treatment in Rheumatoid arthritis patient?

Popliteal cyst excision and synovectomy.

What is the treatment if the patient has associated findings for DVT?
OR
What is the treatment in suspected DVT patient?

Ruptured popliteal cyst may mimic DVT—must do ultrasound of the region to find if the sac is ruptured, and treat for DVT.

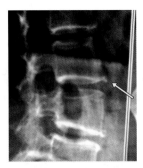

This 50-year-old post menopausal lady came with pain in her back.
What is the typical finding in the disc space?

Cod fish disc space (biconvex).

What is the possible diagnosis?

Osteoporosis.

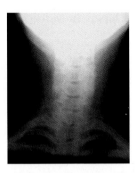

This is a 30-year-old lady who has pain in her little finger and ring finger.
You need to rule out a cervical rib. How will you identify the last cervical spine in this X-ray?

The cervical transverse processes will point downwards.

The thoracic transverse processes will point upwards.

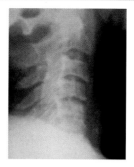

This is an cervical spine radiograph of a 40-year-old man.
What is the finding?
Loss of lordosis—in fact kyphosis.

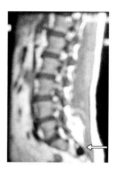

What is this investigation?
MRI.

What one area is difficult to assess by imaging of this region?
Lateral recess lesions.

What is possibly the pointed structure?
Cyst of nerve sheath—usually need conservative treatment only (Tarlov cyst).

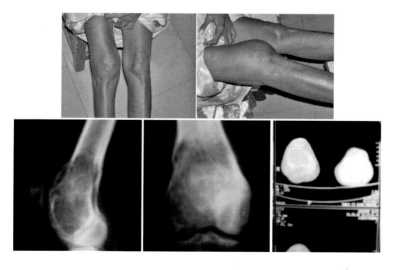

This thirty year old had pain and swelling near her right knee. She had pain on weightbearing. Her X-ray and CT Scan are given. What is the possible diagnosis?

GCT of distal femur.

What is the cell of origin of GCT?

Unknown.

How will you confirm the diagnosis?

Presence of giant cells.

What are the treatment options?

Intralesional

- Curettage
- Adjuvant → Cryotherapy/Cautery
- Bone cement—heat produced kills residual cells
- Packing the defect with bone graft or substitute.

Excision if the bone is expendable. If the lesion is too big—excision and reconstruction. Reconstruction includes arthrodesis, arthroplasty. Radiotherapy for inaccessible lesions.

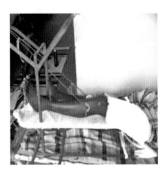

What is the appliance?

The BB splint or Bohler–Braun splint.

How will you select the length of this?

- It has a limb rest with a genu corresponding to the knee.

What are the mistakes in the above picture regarding the use of this appliance?

No stirrup is used.

Weight could not be seen.

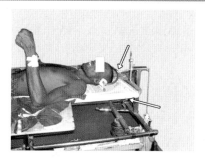

What is this name of this appliance (brown arrow)?
It is called Stryker frame.

What patients are cared in this appliance?
It is used to treat cervical spine injury patients.

What arrangement in this appliance allows the patients to be cared to prevent bed sores?
It has two frames to rotate the patient with a pulley in the upper end.

What is that appliance attached to the patients skull (blue arrow)?
In the above picture the patient is kept in skull tongs traction.

How will you assess the position of the spine in the traction?
Periodic bed side X-rays.

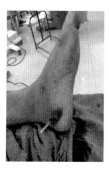

What is the procedure done to this patient?
Calcaneal pin traction

What is the direction of application and why?
Lateral to medial : to avoid peroneal tendon.

What is the indication of this?
For tibial fractures.

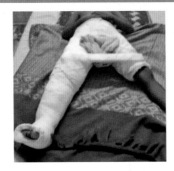

What is this?

One and half hip spica

Which part of the lower limb it addresses?

Used to immobilize hip.

What is the indication of this?

Postoperative cases of fracture neck of femur, dislocated hips in children and femur fractures in children.

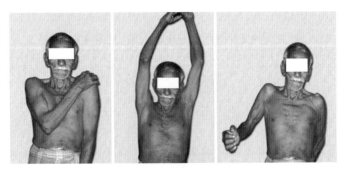

This 60 year old male had a fall landing on his right hand. He has pain in his right shoulder. He can touch the opposite shoulder and also passively lift his shoulder to abduction. He is unable to lift his right upper limb actively.

What is the probable diagnosis?

Rotator cuff tear.

What investigation will non-invasively confirm the diagnosis?

MRI of right shoulder.

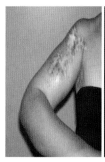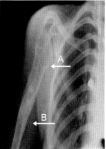

An old osteotomy done for deformity correction in a girl with a congenital condition. What is the possible congenital condition?
Erb's palsy.

What is the position of this shoulder?
Abduction.
Flexion internal rotation.

What is marked as A and B in the X-ray?
A→dysplastic head of humerus.
B→osteotomy site.

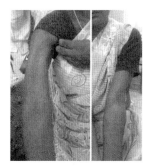

This 40 year old lady had a fall from a two wheeler. This was the picture after 6 months of conservative treatment.
What is the diagnosis?
Malunited humerus fracture

Name one clinical test to confirm the diagnosis?
Transmitted mobility.

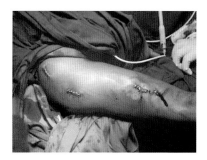

This is a surgery done for right arm region.
What is the possible surgery?
Closed inter locking nailing of humerus fracture.

What is the possible implant?
An humeral interlocking nail.

Where is the entry site?
Proximal entry, with antegrade reaming.

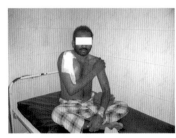 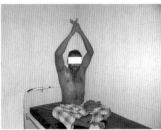

Immediate postoperative status of above case.
What are the movements possible in the immediate postoperative period?
The abduction is done passively in the early postoperative period.

What is your inference regarding the proximal end of the implant with respect to the soft tissue there?
Impingment of rotator cuff by the upper end of the nail is described in books.

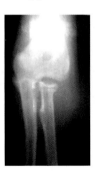

What is wrong with this X -ray?
Capitellum is not in alignment with radial head.

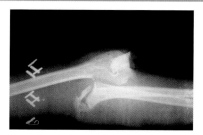

What are the orthopedic injuries?
Total disruption of the elbow complex with fracture olecranon.

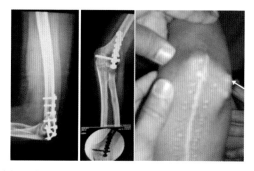

This 16-year-old girl had surgery for distal humerus fracture 1½ years back. You are seeing her X-rays also. What is your diagnosis and advice?
Prominent implants under the skin.
She may be benefitted from implant removal.

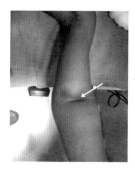

This is the clinical presentation of a 5 year old boy with left elbow injury. This is the finding in the anterior aspect.
What is the possible diagnosis?
Supracondylar fracture.

What is pointed?
Puckering.

What is the possible grade of fracture?
Supracondylar fracture type 3.
Will you try closed reduction in this case?
No.

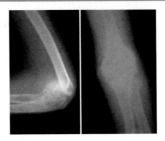

These are X-rays of a 10-year-old boy had this injury and presented after 3 months of routine above elbow plaster in flexion. He presented with an ankylosed elbow and ulnar nerve palsy.

Watch this X-ray? What is peculiarity of this injury?
A case of flexion type of supracondylar fracture

How will you immobilize this fracture?
In extension

How will you treat this condition if this patient presented to you after 3 months?
Extension osteotomy-arthrolysis and anterior transposition of ulnar nerve done in one sitting.

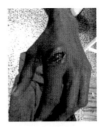

This 25-year-old man had a clean cut injury with a knife. He was not able to actively extend his index finger.

What is the important structure which was cut?
Extensor tendon of index finger

How will you treat him?
Extensor tendon repair.

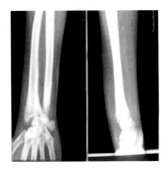

A 45-year-old had pain left wrist, general malaise, loss of appetite and loss of weight. This was his X-ray.

What is the possible diagnosis?

Tuberculosis of wrist.

Which part of the bone is involved?

Lower end of ulna.

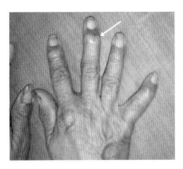

This 60 year old lady had severe pain over the small joints of hands.

What is the lesion pointed?

Heberden's nodules.

What is the diagnosis?

Osteoathritis of interphalangeal joints.

Name one more disease that will specifically affect this joint?

Psoariasis.

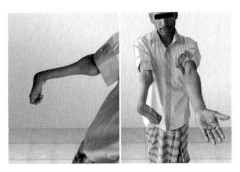

This man had injury to his right elbow and has indigenous massage and tight bandage. He has difficulty in straightening his right side fingers even with other hand. What is the possible diagnosis? What will you do clinically to confirm this? What other examination you will do?

Instruction to the examiner

- The candidate is given a problem of a man who had injury to his right elbow and has indigenous massage and tight bandage. This gentleman also has difficulty in straightening his right side fingers even with other hand. The candidate is asked what is the possible diagnosis? What will he do clinically to confirm this?

- Please see if the candidate checks the extension of the fingers with wrist in flexion and compares the same with the same wrist in extension.
- Please also see if he checks for nerve sensation of median and ulnar nerves.

Please also see if he
- Asks H/o injury, H/o Native treatment and massage
- Elicits Angulation
- Elicits difficulty in using the limb, Rotations restricted, and stiffness of fingers
- Identify atrophic dry and scaly-skin with atrophy of forearm muscles, nail atrophic.

What is the Pathology?
- Sequel to Volkman's ischemia, muscle undergoes ischemic necrosis and replaced by fibrous tissue which causes flexion-contracture of wrist and fingers. There may be peripheral nerve involvement with sensory loss and motor paralysis of hand and forearm.

What are the treatment options?
Passive stretching and splinting
- Soft tissue (muscle) sliding operation (Max Page).
- Shortening of forearm bones—Garre's procedure.
- Carpal bone excision.
- Neurolysis of nerves.

What nerve is commonly involved in this condition forearm? Why?
Median nerve. It runs in the center of the maximum infarcted zone of muscle supplied by anterior interosseous artery. This infarcted muscle can sometimes called as' 'muscle sequestrum' as it is separated by fibrous tissue from the normal muscle.

Questions on ability
What one sign will you elicit?
Volkman's sign.
Wrist and fingers in flexion, looks for sensations ulna/median nerve.
Puts wrist to dorsi flexion of wrist increasing the deformity, In the case of forearm VIC, fingers can be atleast partially extended when the wrist is flexed This is because when the wrist is extended, the shortened muscle tendon unit stretches over the fingers causing extension.

What is Volkman's sign?
The flexion deformities of the fingers are becoming partially correctable with a flexed wrist. The deformities become more pronounced when the wrist is dorsiflexed.

Patient Education can be tested

Advice against massage and native bone setting.

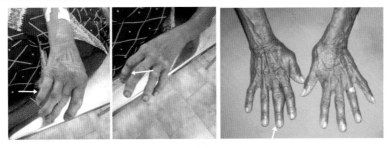

What are the problems of the pointed fingers?
Rheumatoid involvement of small joints.
Swelling of the proximal interphalangeal joints
Ulnar deviation of IP joints.

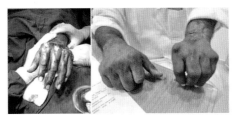

This 50-year-old man had severe stiffness of his left hand finger joints.
What is the surgery done?
Dorsal capsulotomy of MCP joints for a stiff hand.

What is the result?
There is an improved flexion at the metacarpophalangeal joint and interphalangeal joints.

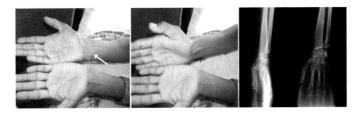

What is the diagnosis?
Prominent ulnar head on the right side in supination → Snaps in pronation.
Negative ulnar variance-with snapping distal ulna.

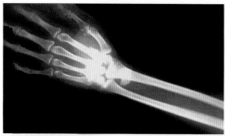

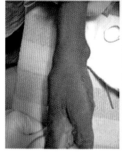 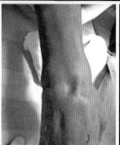 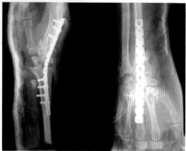

A 45-year-old male was thrown from a two wheeler and does not remember how he landed. These are his clinical pictures of his right wrist with preoperative and postoperative X-rays.

What is the diagnosis?

Wrist dislocation with migration of carpal bones.

What is the bone that is marked with an arrow?

Lunate.

What is the possible cause of the volar prominence marked with an arrow in photos?

Migrated lunate.

What is the treatment done?

Wrist-Fusion Done.

A 60 year old Post Menopausal lady came after indigenous treatment of her left wrist injury. Following are her clinical photographs.

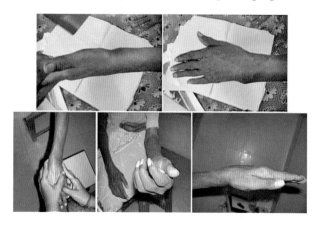

What is the diagnosis?
Malunited Colles fracture.

What is done in figure C?
Level of styloids.

What is seen in figure D?
Stiffness.

What is seen in figure E ?
Dinner-fork deformity.

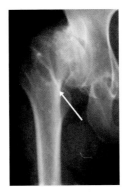

This is an X-ray of a 15 year old boy.
What is the diagnosis?
Slipped upper femoral epiphysis.

What clinical examination is specific for this condition?
Axis deviation.

What will be his general examination finding?
Tall stature, hypogonadism, poor development of secondary sexual characters.

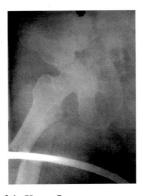

What are the injuries in this X-ray?
Fracture of acetabulum with fracture femur shaft.

How will you manage them?
Fixation of the femur fracture.
ORIF of the acetabulum in one stage.

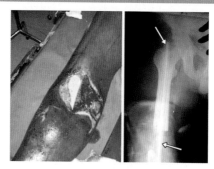

This is a case of open femoral fracture. What is the implant used to fix this?
Antibiotic Laden Acrylic Cement—with a rush nail.

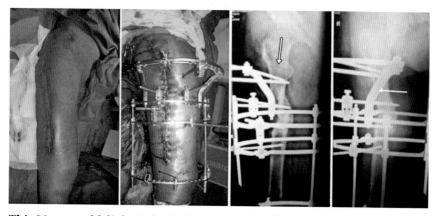

This 30-year-old diabetic had a fracture shaft of femur operated with inter-locking nail. This got infected. He was again operated.
What is this surgery done for him?
Infected fracture femur treated with Ilizaro

What is the pointed structure in lase picture?
Oblique Ilizarov support.

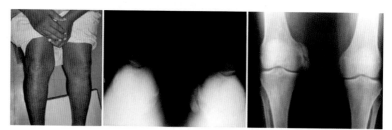

A 50-year-old male came with complaints of pain in the right knee.
What do you see in the X-ray?
Calcification of medial collateral ligament.

Is there any named condition you know?
Pellegrini-stieda disease.

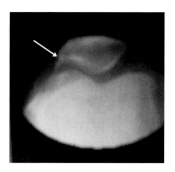

What is this view?
Sunrise view or sky line view of patella.

What is the pointed structure?
Patellar osteophyte.

What is the diagnosis?
Patellofemoral arthiritis.

What will be the difficulty in one activity of daily living?
Climbing stairs.

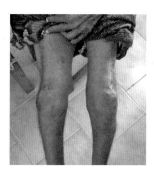

This 52-year-old was born with history of reverse bending of both knees and was delivered by cesarean section. He had surgery done for his both knees when he was 6 months old.

What is the diagnosis?
Congenital dislocation of knees –now after 50 years.

What is the procedure?
Quadriceps lengthening done.

What will be the possible status of both ACL and PCL in this man?
Both ACL and PCL should be deficient.

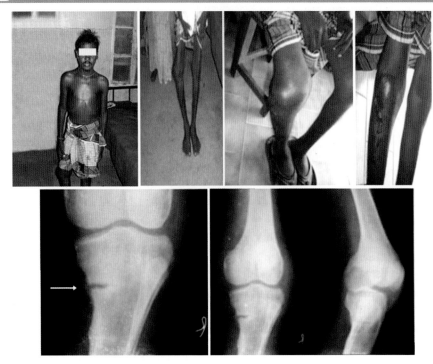

What are the sites involved?
The knee deformity; chest deformity; pigeon chest.

What is the nutritional status of this man?
Stunted growth.

What is the marked lesion in X-ray?
Looser's zone.

What is the possible diagnosis?
Possibility of osteomalacia (rickets).
Genu varus (Rickets).

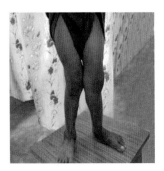

What is this condition?
Genu valgum (Rickets).

What are the measurements useful in assessing the severity of this condition?
Intermalleolar distance.

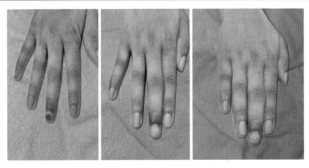

This 30-year-old female had discoloration of the middle fingertip as noted. She had improvement of this with treatment.

What are the investigations that might be done?

Arterial Doppler.

Test for Sickling.

What will be the diagnosis?

Raynaud's disease.

What important diagnosis you should rule out in the neck clinically and radiologically?

Cervical rib.

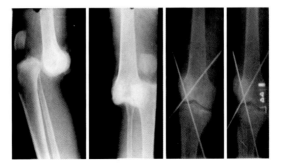

What is this injury?

Dislocation of knee.

How will you manage it?

Closed reduction and stabilization.

Is it an emergency? After all there is no fracture?
What is the most important structure involved?
Popliteal artery is injured and hence it is a surgical emergency what else you will give as a drug?

Heparin.

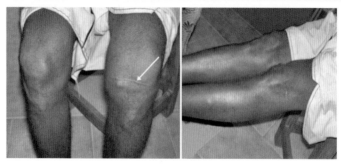

This man had a knee injury and a surgery for the same.

What is the injury?

Comminuted fracture of patella of left side

What is the surgery?

Patellectomy.

What is the postoperative extension?

Extension almost full-postoperatively.

What will be the problem?

or

Can you do total knee replacement in this patient?

It is difficult.

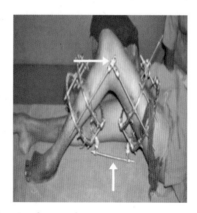

What is the deformity ? What is the joint?

Flexion deformity knee.

What is the treatment?

Treated with Ilizarov.

What are the marked parts with arrows (upper and lower)?

Upper arrow→hinge.

Lower arrow→motor for distraction.

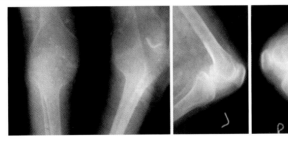

These are the X-rays of knee of an hemophilic.

What is the typical finding in AP view?

The wide intercondylar notch.

Why in the AP view X-ray condyles magnified and distorted?

It is due to associated flexion deformity.

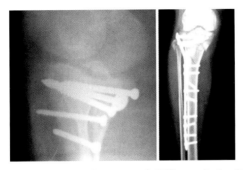

**Two upper tibia fractures were managed differently in different centers.
Which is better?**

Which will allow you early mobilization?

Poor fixation of 1st fracture will result in delayed mobilization. No plate was used.

Second type of fixation shown next allow early mobilization.

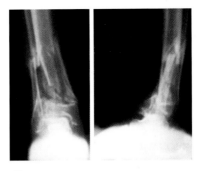

What is the condition?

Comminuted distal tibia fracture and lower end of fibula.

What is the ideal implant if this would be a closed injury?
Minimally Invasive Percutaneous Plate Osteosynthesis for tibia and plating for fibula.

What is the ideal treatment methods if this would be an open injury?
Ilizarov with a foot assembly.

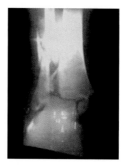

What is the type of injury ?
Pronation -abduction injury ankle.

Why do you say so?
See the lateral cortical comminution in fibula and the avulsion fracture of the medial malleolus.

What is the treatment?
Tension band wiring for medial malleolus and plating for fibula.

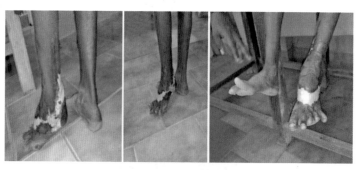

This 20-year-old man had difficulty in moving his left ankle. He had a childhood injury.
Question to the candidate.

What test will you do to confirm this contracture?
Expected outcome-
The candidate asks the patient to do dorsiflexion actively
and confirms by passively attempting the dorsiflexion.

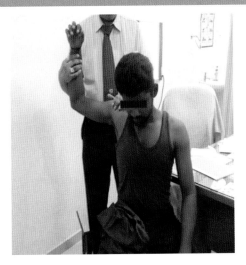

What is movement is done?
The shoulder is abducted and external rotated.

What is this test called?
Apprehension test.

What is the condition if the test is positive?
Recurrent dislocation of shoulder.

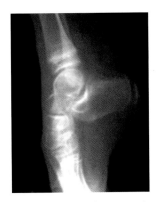

What is the finding in the X-ray of the above patient?
Forefoot–Equinus.

Name the surgery that will address this problem?
Lambrinudi arthrodesis.

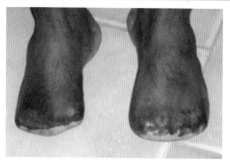

This 40-year-old male had nontraumatic loss of toes
What are the causes?
Arteritis or block of vessels due to atheroma or TAO

What one investigation you will order?
Arterial Doppler of upper and lower limb.

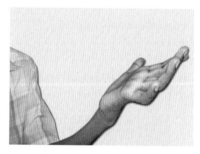

A 25-year-old man came with inability to lift objects with his left upper limb.
O/E this was the inspection- finding

What is the test you will do to find the structure weakened by this causing the deformity?
Power of the intrinsic.

What is the structure which can be substituted for the above weakness?
FDS of ring finger.

This boy had sudden deformity after an elbow surgery. He also had numbness over the little finger and ring finger.
Questions on ability of the candidate.

Check the autonomous region the involved structure?
Greets, Explains test, gets Consent of the patient and Exposes entire both upper limbs.

Explains the test in normal forearm
Asks to tell '1' if the patient feels the sensation.
Then tests the sensation over the affected side ulnar nerve area.

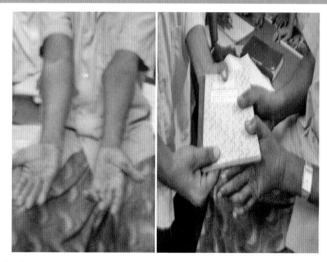

Claw' is the hyperextension of MCP and hyperflexion at IP
ulnar claw – leprosy, ulnar nerve injury.

What is the cause of the deformity seen?
Claw hand-intrinsic minus hand.

What is the autonomous region of the affected structure?
Medial side of the distal phalanx of the little finger.

Why this deformity develops claw hand? (Intrinsic minus)
Intrinsic muscle - Flex MCP and extend the IP.

When intrinsic muscles are paralyzed there is unopposed action of long
flexors and extensors – long flexors – IP flexion; Long extensors – MCP flexion.

What is the treatment of this deformity?
Physiotherapy to keep the joints supple.

Paul Brand I – ECRB

Paul Brand II - ECRL

Total claw – 4 tail transfer

What is the recent tendon used and why?
ECRL is used. Because ECRB was a bulky muscle.

Where in INDIA–pioneering work is done?
Work done in CMC vellore-Prof A.J. Selvapandian.

What is ulnar paradox?
When the nerve lesion is proximal, the deformity is less. When the nerve
lesion is distal, the deformity is more.

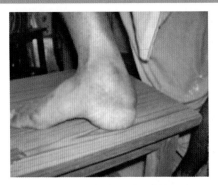

One 50-year-old police man came with prominent swelling over the attachment of tendo calcaneus-with pointed tenderness.

What is the general disease which we must rule out?
Rheumatoid arthritis.

What are the physical modalities of treatment you would advise?
Wax bath.

What additional method you would advise?
NSAIDs.

What will you do in resistant cases?
Excision of the bone in resistant cases.

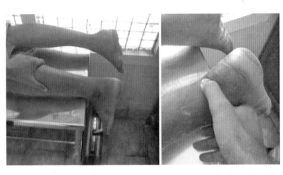

This 50-year-old male had a sudden snapping behind the ankle while jumping.

What is the most possible structure affected?
Closed TA rupture.

How will you diagnose?
What is the test done in figure 1.
Squeeze test.

What is palpated in figure 2?
Palpable gap.

How to diagnose?
H/O sudden give way in 40-50+ age.
The candidate will be watched if he.
palpates a gap in the substance of tendo-Achilles.

Condidate must ask the patient to walk on his toes.

Result → The patient cannot walk on his toes.

Squeezes the calf –and demonstrate no plantar flexion of the foot.

Patient can still attempt a plantar flexion by contracting the long flexors but it is not powerful at all.

What are the other tests for this condition?

Obrien's test needle is introduced into the distal end and then the above test is demonstrated.

What is the another diagnosis which may mimic but is not so devastating?

Plantaris tendon rupture.

Posteromedial and the pain and hematoma is less

More important there is no gap felt over the tendo-Achilles.

What is the tendon that can be of use to augment the TA?

Peroneus brevis.

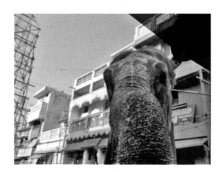

What is this?

This is a temple elephant with his mahout which stopped our car at Kamudhi in South Tamil Nadu.